T0146221

Asklepios, Medicine, and the Politics
of Healing in Fifth-Century Greece

ACKNOWLEDGMENTS

A s with most books, this one, too, has been long in the writing and would not have been possible without the support of many individuals and institutions. Although I single out some for special mention here, I thank you all.

This book began as a Ph.D. dissertation at the University of Texas at Austin under the exceptional direction of Lesley Dean-Jones. Her expertise, critical acumen, and good cheer throughout have shaped this work considerably. She and the other members of my dissertation committee—Erwin Cook, Karl Galinsky, Fritz Graf, and Michael White—have continued to support this project in innumerable ways, and to them I extend my deepest gratitude and thanks.

Various institutions have provided grants, fellowships, and other financial support that not only enabled me to complete this project in all its stages but also facilitated interaction with a host of other scholars who enriched this work immeasurably. These institutions include the American School of Classical Studies at Athens (Gorham Phillips Stevens and Harry Bikakis Fellowships), Gustavus Adolphus College, the Loeb Classical Library Foundation (LCLF Grant), Oberlin College (H. Haskell and A. Johnston Alumni Graduate Fellowships), the University of Cincinnati (Margo Tytus Summer Residency Fellowship, with a special note of thanks to Getzel Cohen, director of the Tytus Visiting Scholars Program, for his gracious hospitality), and the University of Texas at Austin (William S. Livingston Graduate Fellowship, University Co-op Society Graduate Fellowship for Research Excellence).

Likewise, the staffs of these institutions have proven indispensable, and I acknowledge in particular Kathie Martin, ILL librarian at Gustavus Adolphus College, and all the very helpful librarians at the University of Texas at Austin (especially Sheila Winchester, Bonny Keyes, and Gina Giovannone), the Blegen Library of the American School of Classical Studies at Athens (especially

Benjamin Millis and Maria Tourna), the Burnam Classical Library of the University of Cincinnati, and the Jean and Alexander Heard Library of Vanderbilt University (especially Ramona Romero). Thank you also to the directors both recent and current of the American School of Classical Studies—James Muhly, Steven Tracy, and Jack Davis—as well as Maria Pilali, assistant to the director of the school, and Bob Bridges, secretary of the school, for their ongoing support and assistance. I am very grateful also to Nikolaos Kaltsas, director of the National Archaeological Museum, Athens, and Charalambos Kritzas, director of the Epigraphical Museum, Athens, for allowing me to examine and publish photographs of objects in their collections, and to Luigi Beschi for allowing me to publish a drawing of his reconstruction of the Telemachos monument.

Parts of this book were presented as papers at annual meetings of the American Philological Association and the Archaeological Institute of America and as talks and seminars at the American School of Classical Studies at Athens, Gustavus Adolphus College, Oberlin College, Vanderbilt University, and Wabash College. I am grateful to those audiences for their interest and feedback.

Very special thanks to my fellow classicists at Gustavus Adolphus College and Vanderbilt University for being the most supportive of colleagues and friends, especially when it came to finding time and resources for this project. Their enthusiasm has been invaluable. Many thanks to the Classics Department at Gustavus also for providing funding towards permission and publication fees, and to Gusties Henry Boeh, Jonathan Peasley, and Alison Rethwisch for their assistance with images and bibliography.

This book owes much to the talents of acquiring editor Michael Lonegro, manuscript editor Anne Whitmore, and the staff of the Johns Hopkins University Press. An anonymous reader for the press provided many helpful suggestions. Many thanks also to Brent Nongbri for reading and commenting on several drafts of this work, recommending bibliography, and cheering me on and to Denise Demetriou, Robert Drews, and David Petrain for, among other generous deeds, providing valuable feedback on portions of the manuscript. All errors are my own.

Special thanks for their expertise and support to Judith Binder, Sandra Blakely, Courtney Bond, Tommye Corlew, Leda Costaki, Joe Day, Leslie Day, Eric Dugdale, Stewart Flory, Pat Freiert, Will Freiert, Kathy Gaca, Janine Genelin, Jim Hankinson, Ann Hanson, Jesper Jensen, Chrys Kanellopoulos, Carol Lawton, Michaelis Lefantzis, Alexandra Lesk, Daniel Levine, Astrid Lindenlauf, Dale Martin, Margie Miles, Scott Newstok, John Oakley, Olga Palagia, Jennifer Palinkas, Matt Panciera, Gil Renberg, Molly Richardson, Kent Rigsby, Jack Sasson, Peter Schultz, Alan Shapiro, Erika Simon, Tim Smith, Dan Solomon, and Barbara Tsakirgis.

Finally, a most hearty thank you to my family, who have tolerated my years of research abroad and have encouraged me throughout.

A deep sense of irony attached to this project when, in the midst of writing about health and healthcare, a medical crisis visited my own life. In May 2006 my mother was diagnosed with pancreatic cancer. Already at the time of diagnosis it had begun to spread to other organs in her body. She decided to undergo chemotherapy in the hope of extending her life. She died just over three months later after a courageous battle and even more courageous and gracious acceptance of her imminent death. It is to the memory of my mother, Mary Jane Wickkiser, an incomparable woman, that I dedicate this book.

We live in a time when the "miracle of modern medicine" provides not only physical relief but also great hope. But it was not medicine that gave my mother ultimate solace and hope as she struggled with cancer; it was her deep faith in God. For her, confidence in a divine force was not at all incompatible with seeking the help of earthly healers. I think this book will show that many ancient people felt the same way.

All translations are my own unless otherwise indicated. The texts of the medical treatises reproduced in this work are those of W. H. S. Jones and Paul Potter in the Loeb Classical Library volumes of Hippocrates. The text of the Epidaurian *iamata* is that of R. Herzog, *Die Wunderheilungen von Epidauros, Philologus* supp. 22.3, Leipzig, 1931. The text of Aristophanes is F. W. Hall and W. M. Geldart, Oxford Classical Texts; the *Iliad* is D. B. Monro and T. W. Allen, Oxford Classical Texts, 3rd edition; the *Odyssey* is T. W. Allen, Oxford Classical Texts, 2nd edition; Plato is J. Burnet, Oxford Classical Texts; and Thucydides is that of H. Stuart Jones and J. E. Powell, Oxford Classical Texts, 2nd edition. The sources of other texts reproduced in this work are indicated in the notes. I make no pretense about following a consistent pattern for the transliteration of Greek words and names; rather, I often opt for spellings I believe to be most familiar in English.

Abbreviations of ancient authors and their works used in this study are those given in the 3rd edition of the *Oxford Classical Dictionary*, edited by S. Hornblower and A. Spawforth (rev. ed., Oxford, 2003); the *Greek-English Lexicon*, edited by H. G. Liddell, R. Scott, and H. Stuart Jones, 9th edition with supplement, Oxford, 1996; or the *Oxford Latin Dictionary*, edited by P. G. W. Glare, Oxford, 1982.

Other abbreviations used in the text:

BMC   *A Catalogue of the Greek Coins.* British Museum, London, 1873–1927.

CA   *Collectanea Alexandrina.* J. U. Powell, ed. Oxford, 1925 (repr. Chicago, 1981).

CAH²   *Cambridge Ancient History*. Rev. (2nd or 3rd) edition. Cam-
            bridge, 1970–.
CIL   *Corpus Inscriptionum Latinarum*. Berlin, 1863–.
DF   *Claudii Aeliani, Epistulae et Fragmenta*. D. Domingo-Forasté, ed.
            Stuttgart, 1994.
DK   *Die Fragmente der Vorsokratiker*. H. Diels and W. Kranz, eds.
            Dublin, 1966–1967.
ICr   *Inscriptiones Creticae*. M. Guarducci, ed. Rome, 1935–1950.
ID   *Inscriptions de Délos*. Paris, 1926–1937.
IE²   *Iambi et Elegi Graeci*, M. L. West, ed. 2nd edition. Oxford,
            1989–1992.
IG   *Inscriptiones Graecae*. Berlin, 1873–.
IGUR   *Inscriptiones Graecae urbis Romae*. L. Moretti, ed. Rome,
            1968–1990.
I.Perg. III *Altertümer von Pergamon*. Band viii.3: *Die Inschriften des
            Asklepieions*. C. Habicht, ed. Berlin, 1969.
KA   *Poetae Comici Graeci*. R. Kassel and C. Austin, eds. Berlin,
            1983–.
Kühn   *Claudii Galeni Opera Omnia*, C. G. Kühn, ed. Hildesheim, 1965.
L.   *Oeuvres completes d'Hippocrate: Traduction nouvelle avec le texte
            grec en regard, collationné sur les manuscrits et toutes les
            éditions*. E. Littré, ed. Paris, 1839–1861 (repr. Amsterdam,
            1973–).
LIMC   *Lexicon Iconographicum Mythologiae Classicae*. Zurich, 1981–.
LP   *Poetarum Lesbiorum Fragmenta*. E. Lobel and D. Page, eds.
            Oxford, 1955 (repr. 1963).
LSJ   *Greek-English Lexicon*, H. G. Liddell, R. Scott, and H. Stuart
            Jones, eds. 9th edition. Oxford, 1996.
ML   *A Selection of Greek Historical Inscriptions to the End of the Fifth
            Century BC*. R. Meiggs and D. Lewis, eds. Rev. edition.
            Oxford, 1988.
MW   *Fragmenta Hesiodea*. R. Merkelbach and M. West, eds. Oxford,
            1967.
Pauly-   *Real-Encyclopädie der classischen Altertumswissenschaft*.
Wissowa   A. Pauly and G. Wissowa, eds. 49 vols. Stuttgart,
            1894–1980.
PECS   *Princeton Encyclopedia of Classical Sites*. R. Stillwell, ed.
            Princeton, 1976.

RAC	*Reallexikon für Antike und Christentum*. Stuttgart, 1950–.
SEG	*Supplementum Epigraphicum Graecum*. Leiden, 1923–.
Syll.[3]	*Sylloge Inscriptionum Graecarum*. 3rd edition. W. Dittenberger, ed. Leipzig, 1915–1924.
TrGF	*Tragicorum Graecorum Fragmenta*, S. Radt, ed. Göttingen, 1999.

Introduction

... and they shouted the famous refrain, "Great is Asklepios!"

Aelius Aristides, Sacred Tales 2.21

The cult of the Greek healing god Asklepios was one of the most popular in all of antiquity. Individuals afflicted with ailments like blindness, deafness, infertility, paralysis, baldness, and even insomnia, among a host of others, traveled to Asklepios' sanctuaries for cures. Here they would sleep, hoping that Asklepios would visit them in a dream in which he would perform a medical procedure or prescribe a regimen for cure. Evidence as various as coins minted with the god's image, statues and votive plaques featuring the god and his worshippers, and inscriptions documenting his cures attest to the popularity of the cult for over a millennium, from about 500 BC to the sixth century AD. At its height, the cult extended across the length and breadth of the Greco-Roman world.

According to mythological tradition, Asklepios was the son of Apollo and a mortal woman and was trained as a doctor by the centaur Cheiron. He first appears in Homer's *Iliad*, where the Greeks fighting at Troy revere him and his sons, also doctors, for their ability to treat difficult wounds. Later authors describe how Asklepios one day brought a dead man back to life, in return for which Zeus struck Asklepios with a thunderbolt and hurled him into Hades. At some point Asklepios was released from Hades and elevated to the ranks of the Olympians as a healing deity. Although details of the tradition vary (e.g., the identity of his mother, the place of his birth, and the identity of the mortal whom he raised from the dead), its focus throughout antiquity remained Asklepios' skill as a doctor, both while mortal and later when deified.[1]

Literary and epigraphic sources recount the experiences of those who visited Asklepios. A typical visit included preparatory bathing at a spring or well and sacrifices at the god's altar, after which those wanting to be healed would sleep somewhere within the sanctuary, either in a covered space like a stoa or under the open sky. While they slept, the god came to the fortunate individuals in dreams in which he cured their illnesses immediately via surgery or drugs or issued a prescription for diet and exercise to be followed once they had awakened. Those cured by the god dedicated gifts in his sanctuaries, often in the form of body parts fashioned from clay, metal, marble, or wood and depicting the afflicted limb or organ, such as eyes, ears, arms, feet, legs, or breasts.

The cult became so popular that, although Asklepios never had a monopoly on divine healing—the Greeks and Romans worshipped many gods and heroes as healers—he far surpassed all others in the duration and geographic range of his appeal. It would take a new cult based on the worship of another divine healer, Jesus, to ultimately close down Asklepios' sanctuaries, and then only by mandate rather than by obliterating popular interest in him.

While formal worship of Asklepios eventually came to an end, the influence of his cult has persisted. Christian healer-saints like Kosmas and Damian, who were doctors by trade, attracted fervent followings; and popular Christian healing centers like Lourdes in France and the Church of Panagia Evangelistria on the Greek island of Tinos still function today much as did sanctuaries of Asklepios, with the sick bedding down to wait for a cure. Even apart from the tradition's effect on religious healing, some medical associations, including the World Health Organization, continue to feature on their seals Asklepios' iconographic trademark: a walking staff entwined by a serpent.

Common Perceptions of Asklepios and His Cult

Asklepios' appeal extends also to the groves of academe, where he has attracted the attention of scholars of magic, religion, medicine, and dreams since the late nineteenth century, about the time when the earliest archaeological explorations of his sanctuaries got underway.[2] The cornerstone of scholarship on Asklepios and his cult remains Ludwig and Emma Edelstein's monumental two-volume work published in 1945 (reprinted in 1998). The first volume, compiled by Emma Edelstein, contains ancient literary and epigraphic testimonia for the god and his cult arranged by topic, while the second volume, by Ludwig Edelstein, offers a lengthy discussion based on the testimonia.

So influential has this work been on subsequent interpretations of Asklepios' cult that it is important to note some of its limitations. First, it focuses on textual remains to the virtual exclusion of all other types of evidence. The foreword to the 1945 edition, written by Ludwig Edelstein's colleague Henry Sigerist, explains that Edelstein based his interpretation of the cult on literary evidence because of the seeming impossibility of dealing with both material and literary evidence in one work.[3] This limited focus continues in the second volume, where an occasional reference to a coin or statue illustrates a point derived from literary sources.

While the Edelsteins' work remains invaluable to all scholars of Asklepios, any sound analysis of the cult must address both material and literary remains. This has become increasingly true as a wealth of material has been excavated from sanctuaries of Asklepios in the past century and into the new millennium. To ignore this evidence would be to ignore critical aspects of and interpretive windows onto the cult. Scholarship since the Edelsteins' has redressed this shortcoming, as exemplified most recently in the detailed studies by Jürgen Riethmüller, who catalogued the material and literary remains of the cult sanctuary by sanctuary across the ancient world, and by Milena Melfi, who analyzed the god's sanctuaries in Greece in light of recent discoveries.[4]

Second, although Ludwig Edelstein, a scholar of ancient medicine, points to many affinities between mortal physicians and Asklepios, he nevertheless views the cult as "irrational" in contrast to "rational" Greek medicine.[5] This view is not unique to him; it had already been propagated in the nineteenth century by Sir James Frazer. In his epic-long *The Golden Bough*, published in revised and ever-expanding editions from 1890 to 1951 (the first edition of two volumes grew to thirteen by the third edition), Frazer posited an evolution from magic to religion to science that implied a progression from irrational to rational.[6]

Frazer's model proved highly influential. In *The Greeks and the Irrational*, published in 1951, E. R. Dodds forced the cult of Asklepios into Frazer's evolutionary model. Here Dodds spoke of the cult as a "regression" from rationalism and wondered how the Greek mind of the fifth century BC could simultaneously honor the "medical reptile" Asklepios and witness "some of the most austerely scientific of the Hippocratic treatises."[7] For Dodds, Asklepios' cult, full of magic and miracle, occupied the irrational end of an axis at whose other end sat Greek medicine. But if such a stark dichotomy in fact existed, Dodds failed to consider how the Hippocratics themselves could claim the patronage of and even descent from the so-called medical reptile. Dodds created a divide for which we have no evidence at the time. (As documented in his 1977 autobiography, Dodds himself seems to have questioned the rigidity of the categories "rational" and "irrational" in his own experience with the occult, which he believed occupied a "disputed territory between science and superstition."[8]) Moreover, as Helen King observes, casting the medical revolution of fifth-century Greece as a move from religion to science—and, I would add, viewing religion and science as inherently opposed—ultimately tells us more about ourselves and about our own conceptual categories than about the fifth century.[9] And yet, the conceptual framework of rational medicine versus irrational Asklepios cult continues to govern many studies of Asklepios.[10]

Scholars in other fields have begun to question the validity of this dichotomy. For example, Patricia Miller's 1994 study of ancient dreams demonstrates that the Greeks and Romans did not consider dreams irrational. Her conclusions are critical for understanding the nature of Asklepios' cult inasmuch as scholars have long pointed to dreams as a prime indicator of the cult's irrationality.[11] Likewise, Stanley Tambiah's 1990 analysis of magic, science, and religion as interpretive categories conditioned by different cultures and times calls into question their relative definitions and demonstrates in turn how various concepts of rationality have shaped these categories. So, too, does Thomas Harrison's 2006 discussion of "religion" and "rationality" in ancient Greece, where Harrison argues, contra Dodds, that "Greek religious experience . . . is eminently rational." Similarly, G. E. R. Lloyd, one of the most prolific and engaging writers on the relationship between science and the divine in ancient Greece, maintains that marking a sharp divide between "rational science" and "irrational magic" is impossible, given overlap between the methods and explanations of both types of practitioners.[12]

Relevant to Ludwig Edelstein's acceptance of the rational versus irrational divide is his comparison of the cult of Asklepios to Christianity (most evident in a section entitled "Asclepius and Christ"), a move that reinforces the supposed irrationality of the cult in contrast to medicine (rational science).[13] Such an analogy is anachronistic and misleading not only for the first half-millennium of the cult's history, which came before the birth of Jesus, but also for several centuries beyond, when what would become known as Christianity was a struggling movement (even this noun is generous, if not inaccurate), unlike the powerful, organized institution Edelstein adduces. This comparison, moreover, results in questionable conclusions. For example, Edelstein declares that Asklepios' sanctuaries were charitable institutions along the lines of "Christian hospitals and poorhouses."[14] Not only were Christian hospitals and poorhouses a later development of Christianity, but Asklepios' cures were neither charity nor even inexpensive alternatives to other forms of healthcare. An individual wishing to be healed had first to contribute specified amounts of money and other offerings to the god, as we know from inscriptional and literary evidence.[15]

This likening of Asklepios' cult to Christianity has generated a further problematic view of the cult: that it served the needs of private individuals but not the needs of the state. It is widely accepted that Greek and Roman cults played a role in domestic and foreign policy (the Roman practice of *evocatio*, of inviting an enemy state's god to abandon her homeland in favor of Roman residence and citizenship, is but one of the most obvious examples).[16] The cult of Asklepios, however, is regarded consistently as functioning fully apart from what we would call politics. For example, in his discussion of the ease with which cults were transferred, J. K. Davies states in the *Cambridge Ancient History* that "[i]n Greece the instigators were nearly always tyrants or whole communities and the purpose nearly always overtly political. Of course there were exceptions, the most famous and best-documented being perhaps the introduction of the cult of Asclepius to Athens in 420/19 B.C., where no strictly political dimension is visible." And Robert Garland, in *Introducing New Gods*, proclaims, "Of all the cults [investigated in this book] up till now, that of Asklepios stands alone in lacking any apparent political dimension whatsoever."[17]

This interpretive model advanced by Edelstein seems to sit squarely atop the post-Enlightenment church-state dichotomy (or better: Christianity versus state dichotomy). Viewed through Christianizing lenses, Asklepios' cult may appear to operate on a different, indeed less banal plane than other pagan cults mired in the muddy waters of petty power politics; as a Christlike healing god, Asklepios simply would not dirty his hands with such matters. But as we shall see, Asklepios did in fact play a significant role in state affairs. Nor should this surprise us given that "religion" is a category anachronistic to the ancient world. Gods, festivals, sacrifices, prayer, and the like, which we as the heirs of post-Enlightenment ways of thinking collect and analyze as a system discrete from the rest of culture, were in fact part and parcel of every aspect of ancient life, including the functioning of the state, as scholars of religion have been discussing for decades. Wilfred Cantwell Smith's 1963 study of the history of the term "religion," for example, remains useful even as subsequent studies have enriched the dialogue.[18]

Classicists, too, are becoming more aware of the fallacy inherent in talking about ancient religion as if such a discrete entity existed. Jason P. Davies in his 2004 book *Rome's Religious History*, writes, "It may well be that the very idea of religion as a category is in itself misinformed and simply a further legacy of

Christianity. Not all cultures even recognise it as a distinct phenomenon."[19] Still other classicists are attempting to move the discussion in new directions by urging us to understand, in rather stark terms, that the influence between Greek and Roman states and the gods was far from superficial. In a recent and at times provocative analysis of the importance of the Delphic oracle to Athenian democracy, for example, Hugh Bowden makes the bold claim that, "[i]n modern discussions, 'democratic' or more properly perhaps 'Western democratic' regimes are assumed to be liberal, individualist, capitalist and secularist. Democratic Athens was none of these things." He goes on to discuss ways in which the relationship between Athenians and their gods was significant to the polis.[20]

Related to this dichotomy is yet another that is prominent in scholarship: public cult versus private cult. Although the terms are often left undefined, it seems that what is most often meant by "private cult" is that the cult was established and/or controlled by an individual or group rather than by the state. Asklepios' cult broadly, and more particularly his sanctuary in Athens, is often considered an example of a private cult. Sara Aleshire's insightful work on the Athenian Asklepieion is frequently cited for proof that the cult was private, at least until the middle of the fourth century BC. Aleshire's argument, however, rests upon her interpretation of the shift from a lifetime priesthood to an annually rotating one beginning ca. 350 BC.[21] The lack of any inventory inscriptions before ca. 350 must be her main (albeit unstated) proof, since she defines a "state cult" as "one where the Athenian demos and boule, either directly or through their agents, exercise some supervision over the presence and distribution of the votives dedicated in a sanctuary."[22] This argument ex silentio overlooks the possibility that earlier inventory lists existed but have not been recovered. That the priesthood became annual, moreover, does not indicate much at all about state involvement in the cult either before or after 350. Finally, in a cult where individuals meet the god one-on-one in a healing encounter, it is logical that dedications by individuals dominate the evidentiary record, but this does not mean that the state had no involvement in or control over the cult.

Recent studies, furthermore, have argued that no cults in ancient Greece, especially in fifth-century Athens, were distinctly private. Even *oikos*, or domestic, cults were authorized and regulated by the polis. As Robert Parker observes, household shrines were expected to be open for use by Athenians at large, "thus the antithesis between 'public' and 'private' proves not to be absolute even at its extreme points."[23] And Christiane Sourvinou-Inwood argues that the polis "anchored, legitimated, and mediated all religious activity" in the Classical period.[24] Indeed, the intervention of the Athenian polis in cults and sanctuaries is evident in many fifth-century documents, as Robert Garland has discussed.[25]

Regarding Greek cults of the Classical period, it may thus be better to reject the model of a strict public-private dichotomy in favor of a sliding scale of state involvement. There of course remains a difference between the level of state involvement in a cult like that of Athena Polias on the Athenian Acropolis, and that of Egretes, a local hero, in the same city. In the latter, the state may have merely authorized the cult, while in the former it went so far as to organize civic festivals in the god's honor, levy taxes (tribute) on her behalf, appoint priests, and much more.[26] As we shall see, the cult of Asklepios at Athens in fact resides nearer the Athena Polias, or heavy state-involvement, end of this continuum.

The dichotomies of public-private, church-state, and rational-irrational, prominent in Edelstein and persistent in Asklepios studies since, have driven discussion of the cult into interpretive gridlock. Consequently, despite a wealth of scholarship, major questions about Asklepios' cult remain unanswered, or even unasked.

The Current Project

This study addresses a fundamental question about the development and spread of the cult of Asklepios in the fifth century BC: Why did the cult rapidly expand for the first time only in the fifth century even though Asklepios had been known as a healer since Homer? Scholars have long ascribed the enduring popularity of the cult to its personal appeal, especially among societies ravaged by war and plague, as was Greece in the fifth century. Most explanations for the cult's fifth-century expansion, therefore, include some variation of the following causal sequence: widespread disenchantment with the traditional pantheon as the Peloponnesian War and great plague struck; the need for a healing god to treat those suffering plague; growing tension and insecurity as the dominant powers of the period shifted during the course of the war; and the resulting acceptance of "the irrational" coupled with the desire for more personal attention from a gentle god who would care in person for each individual worshipper.[27] However, there has been no convincing explanation as to how or why these particular wars and plagues, and not the other periods of warfare and plague that addled the ancient world, suddenly produced great interest in the cult.

Asklepios' appeal in the fifth century did indeed owe much to his ability to heal. Accounts from Epidauros dating to this time indicate that individuals traveled long distances to be cured of various maladies (striking, by the way, is the absence of plague from these and all other contemporary accounts of Asklepios' cures). But since Asklepios was known as a healer before the fifth century and these same maladies were typical of all periods of Greek history, the evidence raises the question, why now? What about the fifth century drove the sick to consult Asklepios? And why did they turn to Asklepios as opposed to other healing gods?

The first part of this study, Chapters 1–3, proceeds under the assumption that the rational-irrational dichotomy is problematic in antiquity. I argue that the rapid rise in interest in Asklepios derived directly from contemporary developments in medicine. Side-by-side examination of evidence from ancient medicine and Asklepios' cult elucidates important points of contact and even influence between the two: individuals unable to receive treatment from their doctors could go instead to the doctor-god and divine patron of physicians, Asklepios.

Chapter 1 reviews the development of Greek medicine and demonstrates that fifth-century medical treatises advise doctors to turn away patients suffering incurable (mainly fatal and chronic) ailments. In Chapter 2 I look at what sorts of alternatives these same treatises condone for patients who must be turned away and argue that, although overt in their condemnation of most forms of healing, they never criticize or question healing by the gods. Such tacit acceptance of divine healing occurs alongside the rapid expansion of Asklepios' cult, which the latter part of this chapter reviews. In Chapter 3 I argue that the phenomenon of physicians turning away patients suffering chronic ailments and that of the growing popularity of the cult of Asklepios were directly related. Patients turned away by doctors were likely to seek treatment from the doctor-god and divine patron of physicians, Asklepios, whom ancient testimonia consistently describe as curing chronic ailments, many of which were the same sort doctors claimed to be unable to treat.

Concurrent with the growing number of visitors to Asklepios' sanctuary at Epidauros was the establishment of new sanctuaries of the god in other cities. While many scholars have tried to account for the latter by pointing to Asklepios' appeal to ailing individuals, the evidence in the case of Athens, whose importation of Asklepios is well-documented, indicates that the situation was more complicated than heretofore recognized. The second part of this study, Chapters 4–6, sets aside the church-state and public-private dichotomies to explore why Athens, one of the largest and most powerful Greek cities of the fifth century, imported Asklepios from Epidauros in 420 BC.

While the god's appeal to ailing individuals certainly influenced Athens' decision to import the cult, other factors appear to have played an equally if not more immediate role. The reexamination, in Chapter 4, of the so-called Telemachos monument, our primary evidence for the importation, demonstrates that its inscription, which has long been read as describing a single man's efforts to found the sanctuary, contains ample indication that Athens as a civic entity had a vested interest in importing the god. Chapter 5 begins with a questioning of the traditional view that the great plague of 430–426 BC prompted the importation. Next, drawing on recent observations about the impact of ritual upon culture in both its spatial and temporal dimensions, I analyze where the cult was positioned within the topography and festival calendar of Athens. I do so under the assumption that these points in space and time are key indicators of the nature of Athenian interest in the cult.[28] I look in particular at the integration of the cult into the Acropolis and its slopes, and into the cults of Dionysos Eleuthereus and Eleusinian Demeter. Given the marked associations of these loci with Athenian empire in 420, I propose that the importation of Asklepios be understood in relation to Athenian aspirations about its empire. Chapter 6 returns to the historical context of the importation to argue that Athens imported Asklepios from Epidauros to forge an alliance with a city critical to Athenian success against Peloponnesian aggression.

Analysis of the cult in relation to both medicine and politics affords a fuller and more complex understanding of why the fifth century in particular was a defining moment for this cult. The arguments and conclusions in the following pages are by no means intended to provide a complete explanation for Asklepios' appeal; rather, my hope is to modify and expand traditional explanations for the early development of a cult that proved attractive to worshippers for more than nine hundred years and that remains relevant to the medical profession two and a half millennia later.

CHAPTER ONE

From Practice to Profession

The Development of Greek Medicine from the Bronze Age to the Fifth Century BC

In the absence of health, wisdom cannot display itself, art is not evident, strength is unexerted, wealth is useless, and speech powerless.

Herophilos of Keos, Dietetics, *as quoted by* Sextus Empiricus, Against the Mathematicians 11.50

The Greeks, from at least the Bronze Age on, had many ways to heal the human body: these included prayer, sacrifice, incantations, philters, amulets, drugs, poultices, bandages, and surgery, to name but a few. Most people probably had some basic healing knowledge,[1] but they could also consult healers with more specialized and advanced knowledge, such as magicians (μάγοι), root-cutters (ῥιζοτόμοι), priests (ἱερεῖς), doctors (ἰατροί), doctor-prophets (ἰατρομάντεις), purifiers (καθάρται), and drug vendors (φαρμακοπῶλαι). In practice, no rigid lines separated the various means of healing; different practitioners used different combinations of these elements. Drugs, for example, were frequently used by magicians, doctors, root-cutters, and drug vendors, but in various combinations with other methods. The term ἰατρομάντις itself suggests an overlap, in addition to a dichotomy, between the methods of the iatros, or doctor, and those of the mantis, prophet.[2]

Despite the potential overlap in method, certain types of healers tended to employ certain modes of healing more often than others. Magicians and priests, for instance, brought about cures by communicating with and influencing deities who were thought to have caused illness, and thus they often employed methods like prayer, sacrifice, and incantations to effect communication with the divine.[3] The doctor more commonly employed bandages, surgery, drugs, poultices, and the like to heal the body without divine intervention.

This chapter surveys the early development of healing practices whose efficacy can be explained without reference to the intention of any divine being.[4] The Greeks had no label for this type of healing—at least not at first. They did consistently distinguish the *iatros* (doctor) as a type of healer who avoided methods like amulets and prayer that were meant to influence the will of the gods, and in the fifth century they coined the term *iatrike*, medicine, to describe the healing practiced by doctors. Thus, for the sake of convenience, I shall refer to such practices as "medicine" or "medical," although they were never the exclusive purview of doctors, nor did they spring suddenly into use in the fifth century.[5] The practice of medicine was not entirely dissociated from the divine; for example, doctors claimed descent from Asklepios and swore to the gods to uphold certain standards (the famous Hippocratic Oath).

The presence of this so-called medical healing in the early historic and even prehistoric record demonstrates that what later became formally known as medicine represents a refinement, categorization, and further professionalization of methods employed by all sorts of healers since at least the Bronze Age. The affinities between doctors and Asklepios that made the god such a fitting patron of the medical profession extend back at least to Homer and the first descriptions of doctors in epic poetry.

The Bronze Age and Homer

Medical healing left traces in Bronze Age Greece. At Pylos, Knossos, and Mycenae, for example, clay tablets record spices that may have been used as drugs for healing. These include *ep-i-ka* (ebiscus), *ko-ri-a-da-na* (coriander), *ka-na-to* (safflower), and *ko-ro-ki-no* (saffron). Skeletal remains indicate that certain ailments, like fractures, were treated by the immobilization of bones with splints. A Mycenean tomb dating to 1450 BC has yielded drills, scalpels, forceps, and grinding stones for the preparation of drugs. And a tablet listing various occupations mentions the word *i-ja-te* (related to the later Greek word *iatros*, which first appears in Homer). The same word may also appear in an inscription on a Minoan pithos dated to ca. 1550 BC.[6]

Homeric epic provides the earliest extant description of Greek healing methods in the Archaic period (ca. 750–500 BC). Greek literature begins with a disease: at the opening of the *Iliad*, the Greeks encamped at Troy suffer from a plague brought on by the god Apollo. They believe the only way to rid themselves

of the plague is to appease the deity who sent it by means such as prayer, purification, and animal sacrifice.[7] In the *Iliad* this plaque has a divine causation
and a divine cure, but reliance on the divine as an aid to healing is not limited
to disease. In Book 5, when a stone hurled at the Trojan warrior Aeneas crushes
his hip socket and rips through two of his tendons, Apollo whisks him from
the battlefield to the care of Leto and Artemis. Apollo's mother and sister heal
the wound, it would appear, simply by their divine presence (*Il.* 5.445–448). The
role of the divine in human health, as in all aspects of human existence, is central to this epic.

In addition to recounting the prevalent role of the divine, the *Iliad* often describes healing, especially of wounds, as occurring without recourse to prayers,
incantations, or other attempts to communicate with the gods. When an arrow
lands deep in Eurypylos' thigh in Book 11 and "sweat flowed in streams from
his head and shoulders, and dark blood poured from his gruesome wound," the
Greek warrior beseeches his comrade Patroklos: "Save me, lead me back to my
black ship, and cut the arrow from my thigh; wash the black blood from it with
warm water, and spread it with gentle herbs." Patroklos agrees to help Eurypylos: "Patroklos stretched him out and cut the sharp arrow from his thigh with a
knife, and washed the dark blood with warm water, and having crushed a bitter,
pain-slaying root (ὀδυνήφατον ῥίζαν) in his hands, applied it to the wound. The
root stopped all his pains; the wound dried and the blood stopped flowing" (*Il.*
11.804–848). All of the wounds treated by human healers in the epic are treated
in much the same way, with poultices of drugs and often bandages.[8]

Even certain wounds suffered by the gods—for instance, by Hades and Ares
in Book 5—are treated by medical means rather than prayers or magical touch,
although their healer Paieon is himself a god. When Paieon heals Hades, he
spreads pain-slaying herbs (ὀδυνήφατα φάρμακα) on the wound (*Il.* 5.395–402).
When Paieon heals Ares, moreover, Homer makes an empirical observation
about the effect of the drugs: they are compared to a natural physical process—
to the quick curdling of milk when fig juice is added (*Il.* 5.902–904).[9] This is
the first example of what might be called scientific simile, and it indicates that
medical methods could be distinguished from other forms of healing, like incantations.[10] It seems that these methods were so well known and, in the case
of battle wounds, so effective that the gods themselves were sometimes envisioned as using them.

The typical Iliadic warrior must have had basic first aid skills, especially after fighting for ten years at Troy. Some warriors, like Patroklos, acquired
greater healing knowledge through special training. Patroklos learned to heal

from Achilles, who had been taught by the centaur Cheiron (Il. 11.831–832). Patroklos' treatment of Eurypylos demonstrates his advanced skill: he knows how to excise bits of metal weapons lodged in the body, cleanse wounds, and apply poultices of drugs to ease the pain and coagulate the blood.

Yet Patroklos is not the most skilled healer on the Homeric battlefield. The best healers are doctors, who are summoned in the most critical cases. In Book 4, panic descends on the Greek camp when an arrow lodges in the belly of the Greek king Menelaus. His brother Agamemnon, wringing his hands, reassures him that he will get the best healthcare possible: "A doctor will treat the wound and apply drugs to stop the dark pains" (Il. 4.190–191), and Agamemnon sends a messenger to summon the doctor Machaon. Likewise, when Eurypylos is wounded in Book 11, his first instinct is to look for a doctor; only when he realizes none is available does he turn to Patroklos (Il. 11.833–836).

Homer describes in great detail how the doctor Machaon treats Menelaus' wound: first he slides the barbed arrow out of the warrior's belt; then he undoes several layers of Menelaus' attire to uncover the wound; finally, having sucked the blood from it, he spreads the wound with drugs (Il. 4.193–218). Homer elsewhere calls doctors "those of many drugs" (πολυφάρμακοι, Il. 16.28; also Eustath. Il. 11.833), since a doctor's treatment of wounds so often involved drugs. While the healing Homer describes is mainly surgical, it may also have included the fighting or prevention of infection, a prime threat on any battlefield.[11] But nowhere in Homer does a doctor use modes of healing meant to influence the will of the gods.

Homer mentions only three doctors by name: the brothers Machaon and Podaleirios and their father, Asklepios. This is the earliest evidence of Asklepios, and here he appears to be merely a mortal doctor; there is no mention of divine ancestry. Nevertheless, he is esteemed for his healing skill: he is twice called a noble healer (ἀμύμων ἰητήρ, Il. 4.194, 11.518). Likewise his son Machaon, when wounded in Book 11, inspires the warrior Idomeneus to proclaim as he hurries to save Machaon and his healing talents, "A doctor is a man worth many other men (ἀνὴρ πολλῶν ἀντάξιος ἄλλων) when it comes to cutting out arrows and sprinkling on soothing herbs" (Il. 11.514–515).[12]

The repetition of "many" in this phrase and in "those of many drugs" (Il. 16.28) suggests that the Homeric doctor is quantitatively different from ordinary people inasmuch as he possesses the combined knowledge of many men. But the difference is also qualitative: by knowing more, he thereby also knows better how to heal. Moreover, Homer distinguishes doctors from others by specialized training. As with any other craft, the procedures and skills of doctors had to be learned. The centaur Cheiron is said to have given Asklepios drugs to use (φάρμακα, Il. 4.217–219), just as he also taught (ἐδίδαξε, Il. 11.830–832) the hero Achilles to heal. The father-son relationship between Asklepios and Machaon and Podaleirios suggests also a familial model for the training of some doctors, typical of most crafts in antiquity.

Like the Iliad, the Odyssey attests to the demand for doctors: people across the endless earth seek them along with prophets, builders, and poets (Od. 17.383–386).[13] The grouping of doctors with prophets, builders, and poets, agents who produce, suggests the efficaciousness of doctors; others could not provide the same type of healing, or at least not to the same degree of quality. And Eumaeos in the Odyssey speaks of the doctor as a δημιοεργός, a craftsman, or literally "worker of the people" (Od. 17.383–385).

In Homeric tradition, then, medical healing plays a prominent role. It is the most common form of healing on the battlefield and its best practitioners are doctors, who are much respected for their particular skills. These skills constitute a craft that must be learned and, in some cases, is handed down from father to son.

Between Homer and Hippocrates

Evidence for medical healing is sparse until the early sixth century BC, due mainly to the fact that evidence for nearly everything is sparse in this period. But by the early sixth century, the poetry of Solon attests to the respect extended to doctors and their distinction from other healers. In his prayer to the Muses, Solon lists doctors among various occupations of men:

> . . . others are doctors and have the task of Paieon of the many drugs. For these men there is no end of labors, since very often a small discomfort becomes a great suffering. Nor could anyone alleviate it even by administering gentle drugs. But it is also the case that a doctor might quickly heal with his hands one overcome by wretched, painful illnesses. (Solon, IE² Fr. 13.57–62)[14]

Solon characterizes doctors by their use of drugs and other physical intervention (ἀψάμενος χειροῖν, a phrase that could refer to any number of procedures, such as surgery or the application of cupping instruments).[15] Moreover, he recognizes doctors for their ability to quickly heal dire cases when, as he elaborates, Fate (Μοῖρα) allows.

The organization of medicine seems to have undergone a major development by the early sixth century. According to the epic poet Arktinos, whose Sack of

Troy dates to the seventh or sixth century BC, the doctor Machaon (here described as the son of Poseidon) mainly treated wounds while his brother Podaleirios treated internal disorders, including the madness of Ajax (Schol. ad Il. 11.515; Eustath. Il. 11.514). This split points to a differentiation between internal and external healing that is absent in Homer, although the Iliad's omnipresent demand for battle-wound management may simply have eclipsed any description of internal healing.[16]

Beginning in the sixth century BC, medicine shared a discourse and vocabulary, theories and ideas with early teachings of philosophy.[17] According to Aristotle, Thales, born ca. 625 BC in Miletos, founded Ionian science (Arist. Metaph. 983b20 = DK 11A12). As the purported founder of a new way of thinking about the world, Thales looked to causes other than the gods to explain certain events. For example, he explained the phenomenon of an earthquake not in terms of Poseidon's wrath causing him to shake the earth with his trident but in terms of the sometimes-violent movement of the waters on which, he postulated, the earth floated (Sen. Q Nat. 3.14 = DK 11A15).[18]

At the same time, the function and malfunction of the human body were also being described in terms other than godly involvement. By the late sixth and early fifth century, Alcmaeon, a philosopher and possibly also a doctor from the Greek colony of Croton in Magna Graecia, attributed the health of the human body to the balance ($\mathit{i\sigma o\nu o\mu i\alpha}$) of four elements: hot, cold, wet, and dry (Aëtius 5.30.1 = DK 24B4).[19] He also advanced theories on the physiology of the body, such as the brain being the seat of the intellect and semen being the main constituent of the brain.[20] Alcmaeon relied heavily on empirical observation in order to describe the functioning of the sense organs of the human body. For example, he said that hearing takes place through the ears because they contain a void that resounds; sound is produced in the cavity and echoed by the air.[21] These arguments based on reason and empirical observation are similar to the types of arguments and observations made in the earliest medical treatises.

The complex influences of medicine on philosophy and vice-versa are frequently perceived and described by scholars only in terms of the influence of philosophy on medicine. It is more likely, however, that philosophers would have extrapolated from observations of the microcosm (i.e., the human body) to the macrocosm.[22] Just as doctors were thinking of healing as independent of the intention of specific gods (as attested in Homer), philosophers were mapping similar patterns and ideas onto the workings of the cosmos. That the direction of influence flowed, at least in part, from medicine to philosophy is supported by the early publication of medical treatises. Some of the extant treatises have been dated to the early fifth century and may reflect still earlier tradition.[23]

Moreover, certain geographic areas, including Ionia and Magna Graecia, were associated with both natural philosophy and medicine from an early period.[24] Centers of medical thought, if not also training, developed by at least the sixth century BC. Croton, in Magna Graecia, was one such center; it was the home not only of Alcmaeon and his predecessor Pythagoras but also of Democedes, a doctor who practiced in the second half of the sixth century and one of the earliest Greek doctors whose name has survived in literature.

Conforming to the description of doctors in the Odyssey, Democedes and his skills were in such demand that he found work at Aegina and Athens, was hired by the tyrant Polykrates of Samos, and was even compelled by the Persian king Darius to treat the king's injured ankle (Hdt. 3.129–130, 132).[25] At Aegina, he surpassed all other doctors despite his lack of equipment (Hdt. 3.131). And in Susa, where his reputation as a doctor brought him to Darius' attention, he feared that discovery of his skills might prevent his ever leaving Persia (Hdt. 3.130). His position in Aegina certainly, and probably also in Athens, was a public position. The city hired him presumably to tend to its healing needs, and thus he is the first attested example of a "public doctor" (often referred to as ἰατρὸς δημοσιεύων or δημόσιος ἰατρός) in Greece.[26] According to Herodotus, his salary increased with each successive post (Hdt. 3.131). Moreover, because of Democedes' skill, Croton acquired a reputation as the home of the best doctors in Greece, with Cyrene taking second place (Hdt. 3.131).

The level of respect, status, and potentially even wealth that a practitioner of medicine could acquire by the late sixth century is evident also from a fragmentary relief, now in Basel, celebrating an unnamed healer (Fig. 1.1).[27] Little is known about the relief, including its original provenance and its purpose (whether grave relief, votive relief, etc.). It depicts two figures: a bearded man seated with a walking staff in his hand, and another, discernible as a younger male despite the relief's poor preservation, standing and facing the seated figure. The posture of the seated figure would become the standard way of depicting doctors in later works of art such as tombstones and rings; the doctor sits on a chair, often to examine a patient in front of him.[28] Cupping instruments, which would come to be associated primarily, if not exclusively, with doctors, appear above the two figures and also hang from the arm of the standing youth. Doctors used cupping instruments to draw sickness carried by humors (fluids like blood and bile) away from the body. After being heated, the

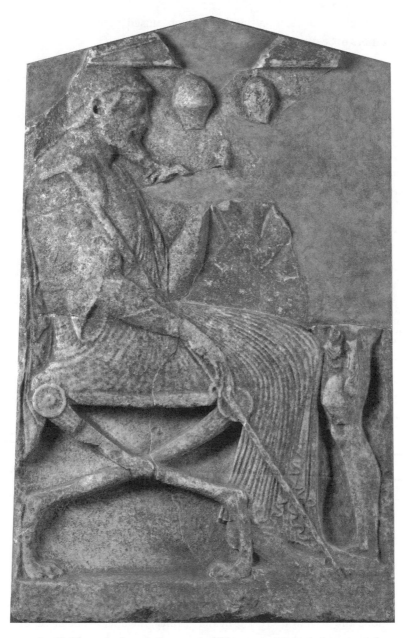

Figure 1.1. A relief from the late sixth or early fifth century BC depicting a seated physician, walking staff resting against his shoulder, facing another figure, poorly preserved. Cupping instruments appear between the heads of the figures. (Antikenmuseum Basel, BS 236. Photo courtesy of the Antikenmuseum Basel und Sammlung Ludwig.)

cups were placed still hot on the skin, which caused a vacuum to develop and the humors to be drawn out towards the skin.[29]

The cupping instruments in the relief, together with the walking staff (symbol of an itinerant lifestyle) and posture of the bearded man, indicate that whoever commissioned the relief specifically intended to portray a doctor. The status and visibility of at least some doctors must therefore have been prominent, and their nature and duties well enough known that a visual shorthand (e.g., cupping instruments, walking staff) could distinguish them from other types of healers.[30]

Another work of art, this from Attica dating to ca. 510–500 BC, celebrates a doctor named Aineas (Fig. 1.2). A painted marble disk designed for a funerary context (possibly to cover an urn or an opening in a tomb through which offerings were received), it bears the inscription: μνῆμα τόδ᾽ Αἰνέο σοφίας ἰατρὸ ἀρίστο ("This is a memorial of the skill of Aineas, best of doctors").[31] The painting, although now badly worn, depicts a bearded man sitting in a chair—the same posture as the doctor in the Basel relief. The epithet "best of doctors" implies that he achieved, or claimed to have achieved, a high level of prestige and renown based particularly on his skill (σοφία).

Figures like the healer on the Basel relief, "best of doctors" Aineas and their more fully documented peer Democedes of Croton demonstrate that some doctors could attain at least as high a level of prominence in the sixth century BC as had their counterparts in Homer.[32] In addition, the demand for skilled doctors was so great that some cities, like Aegina, began paying them for services, and certain areas, among them Croton, became known as centers for medical training and produced some of the finest practitioners of their kind.

Tradition and Change in Fifth-Century Medicine

In the fifth century, these trends continued to develop. A red-figure aryballos of ca. 480 BC, the "Peytel aryballos," depicts a healer at work with as many as six patients to his left and right, all stricken with various maladies like skin irritations and flesh wounds. The healer applies a scalpel to one patient's forearm in the process of letting blood, a procedure identifiable by the basin situated beneath the patient's arm to catch the blood flow (Fig. 1.3).[33] As in the Basel relief, cupping instruments hang above the healer and leave no doubt as to his profession.

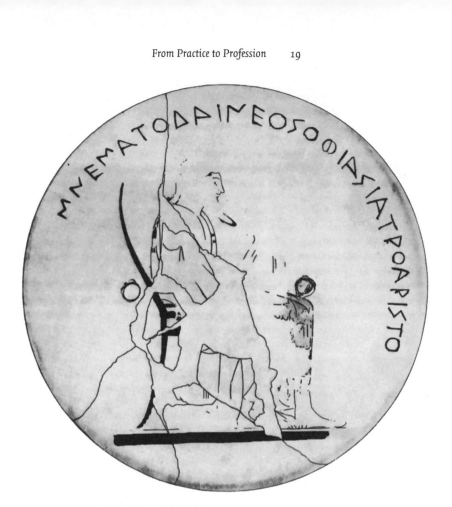

Figure 1.2. Drawing of a painted memorial from the late sixth century BC celebrating the physician Aineas. The inscription reads: "This is a memorial of the skill of Aineas, best of doctors." (National Archaeological Museum, Athens, 93. Drawing by Henry Boeh, after Berger 1970, fig. 17.)

Doctors also appear in literature of the time. In Aristophanes' *Acharnians* of 425 BC, when a man approaches Dikaiopolis for some balm to soothe his sore eyes, Dikaiopolis barks, "Go away, scoundrel. I am not the public doctor" (οὐ δημοσιεύων τυγχάνω, *Ach.* 1030). But according to the play, someone named Pittalos certainly is (1032), and the general Lamakos later asks to be taken with healing hands (παιωνίαισι χερσίν, 1222) to Pittalos. By contrast, in Aristophanes' *Ploutos*, produced in 388 BC, doctors are notable for their unusual absence. The protagonists want to have the god Ploutos, or Wealth, healed of his

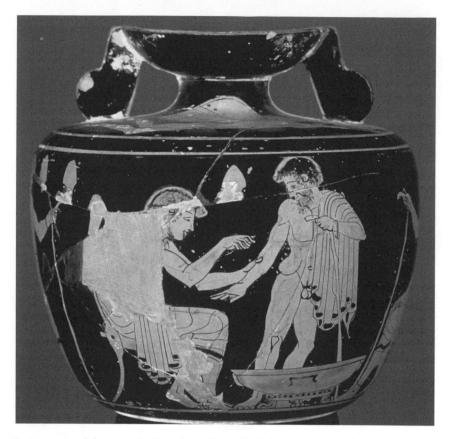

Figure 1.3. A red-figure aryballos of ca. 480 BC depicting a healer bleeding a patient over a collecting basin. A cupping instrument hangs in the background between the two figures. Other individuals (not visible here) stricken with various maladies stand to their left and right. (Louvre, Paris, CA 2183. Photo from Réunion des Musées Nationaux / Art Resource, NY.)

blindness so that his distribution of riches will be more just. They think first to take him to a doctor, but Chremylos cries rhetorically, "Is there a doctor in all the city? There is no pay, and therefore there is no *techne* (skill)" (Pl. 407–408).[34] The fact that a doctor was the first and most obvious resort demonstrates an expectation both of the presence and accessibility of doctors by the early fourth century, a natural result of the growing visibility and acceptance of doctors in the previous century.

Although Democedes is the only known public doctor from the sixth century, literary accounts from the late fifth century attest to annual competitions for the post of public doctor in cities like Athens. Plato's *Gorgias* speaks of these posts and of public physicians generally as something with which Socrates' immediate audience was familiar without explanation.[35] And the discourse which natural philosophy and medicine shared beginning in the sixth century continued to develop in the fifth century with philosophers like Parmenides of Elea, Diogenes of Apollonia, and Empedocles of Akragas, who put forward medical theories. These thinkers continued to coalesce around Ionia and Magna Graecia.[36]

Such threads of continuity not only make it possible to gauge in broad terms the development of Greek medicine since the Bronze Age society presented by Homer but also demonstrate the longevity of the tradition. Much of the evidence points to development as opposed to drastic change. Doctors, men whom the *Iliad* had estimated as worth countless others for their skills, could now receive a formal position and salary as public doctors in some cities. Moreover, their remuneration based on contract or an agreed scale of fees indicates the level of professionalization some had attained, while their depiction in works of visual art like pottery and reliefs points to their status and formal recognition. Meanwhile, a demand for doctors continued to compel many of them to travel, much as Homeric doctors had done.

While the evidence thus points emphatically towards continuity, ancient sources posit a milestone in the development of medicine in the fifth century BC. Change coalesced around the figure of Hippocrates, the best-known doctor in ancient history. Born ca. 460 BC on the island of Kos, Hippocrates was known already by his contemporaries as a famous doctor, referred to simply as "Hippocrates the Koan, one of the Asklepiads" (Pl. *Prt.* 311b–c) and an authority on the relationship between the body and nature (Pl. *Phdr.* 270c). He was considered on a par for his profession with the sculptors Polykleitos and Pheidias and the poet Homer (Pl. *Prt.* 311c–d). Thus even while alive he was considered a paradigmatic representative of his profession.[37]

It is remarkable, given his fame during or shortly after his lifetime, how scant contemporary or near-contemporary references to him are. We have only the two from the whole of Plato and nothing else. It is still more remarkable that Athenians of his own day already thought him an outstanding doctor even though he is not known to have visited Athens.[38]

Hippocrates' reputation grew tremendously as time passed. In the first century AD, the physician Scribonius Largus would call him "the founder of our profession" (*Comp.* 5); Seneca would say that he was the greatest doctor and the founder of medicine (*Ep.* 95.20); and Celsus would eulogize him as "a man most worthy of being remembered, notable for his technical skill and elo-quence" (*De med.* 1.praef.8). By the second century AD, Galen made even these comments seem stingy and lackluster by heaping frequent, hyperbolic praise on Hippocrates in many of his writings.[39] The repeated emphasis on Hippo-crates as "the founder of medicine" reflects the ancient view that he marked the beginning of a new phenomenon. Even modern scholars perpetuate this tradition by referring to Greek medicine as "Hippocratic medicine."

While much of what we know of Hippocrates, and indeed much of what the ancients knew about him, is almost certainly a fabrication, a number of phe-nomena attaching to this figure mark new developments in the area of medi-cine, or ἰατρική (iatrike) as it was called by the fifth century.[40]

Medicine as a *Techne*

The demarcation of a particular type of healing as *iatrike* was motivated by the desire to define medicine as a τέχνη, a skill acquired through learning as opposed to inspiration or some other mode of acquisition (often translated into English more simply as "craft" or "art").[41] A reference in Plato's *Sophist* to Protagoras' writings "on wrestling and the other arts" (περί τε πάλης καὶ τῶν ἄλλων τεχνῶν, *Soph.* 232d–e) indicates the number and diversity of such *technai*, as well as their prominence in discourse. So, too, do the opening words of the Hippocratic treatise *On the Art (Techne)* where the author states that he is re-sponding specifically to those people who make a practice of vilifying *technai* generally (*De arte* 1 = 6.2 L.).[42]

Various disciplines were carving out their own niches as distinct *technai* and many were using treatises to do just that. Rhetoric is one of the most prominent examples of this phenomenon from the last quarter of the fifth century.[43] Much of Plato's *Gorgias*, for example, is an attempt to determine the particular *techne* of rhetoric. One of Socrates' interlocutors in the *Gorgias* is Polus, a teacher and author of a rhetorical treatise called Τέχνη to which So-crates refers (*Grg.* 462b11). Socrates, not persuaded by the arguments Polus has made in his treatise, presses both him and the rhetorician Gorgias fur-ther as to the precise nature of their *techne*. As Gorgias and his followers struggle to name what exactly it is that their *techne* concerns, Socrates declares that rhetoric cannot be a *techne* because, "[i]t cannot give an account of that to which it applies, and therefore cannot name the cause of each" (*Grg.* 465a2–5). His point is that rhetoric can only be a *techne* if one can explain what skill is unique to it.

In the course of trying to get Gorgias and Polus to tell him what rhetoric concerns in particular, Socrates frequently returns to medicine as a prime example of a *techne*, since everyone knows what it deals with: the health of the human body. In fact, it is the first *techne* that Socrates uses as a model in the dialogue (Grg. 448b4–10). It recurs more famously later in the *Gorgias* when Socrates contrasts the *techne* of medicine with the knack (ἐμπειρία) of cookery (ὀψοποιική), which aims not at what is the best for the body but at what is most pleasing to it (Grg. 463c5–466a3).[44] Thus, while rhetoric was still trying to prove itself as a *techne*, medicine was easily recognizable as one. Even the title of the Hippocratic treatise *On Ancient Medicine* (Περὶ ἀρχαίης ἰατρικῆς) suggests the relative age of medicine versus other *technai*.[45]

Medicine and Its Limits

The term *iatrike* is itself indicative of development. It occurs in the literary record for the first time in the fifth century BC, but at exactly what point is a matter of dispute.[46] Herodotus uses *iatrike* to refer to healing practiced by the Egyptians (Hdt. 2.84, 3.129). It also occurs repeatedly in Plato's *Gorgias*, written ca. 385 BC but having a dramatic date roughly in the last quarter of the fifth century. Here it applies to Greek healing, and its use does not appear novel to the dialogue's participants.

The term "iatrike" also appears in medical treatises of the fifth century BC and later that have come down to us under the name of Hippocrates. The corpus of writings collected by Alexandrian scholars and attributed en masse to Hippocrates was understood even in antiquity to have been written by more than one author.[47] Although the names of these other authors became separated from their works, the mere fact that many different people were writing about medicine is indicative of lively discourse on the subject. Moreover, the range of audiences to which the treatises were aimed, from prospective students to those already studying medicine, attests to its widespread interest.[48] These writings of the fifth century helped advance the professionalization of medical healing. Doctors published their own thoughts about the true causes of illness and proper methods of treatment. These writings are invaluable as one of the first windows onto the treatment of nonacute ailments in ancient Greece (especially those contracted off the battlefield). Uncertainty about the dates of the individual treatises makes it hard to say when the term *iatrike* was first used by these authors, but it appears in *Airs, Waters, Places*, generally agreed to be one of the earliest (early fifth century) Hippocratic treatises.

The coining of "iatrike" reified the practice of medicine as something separate from its practitioners and thus as capable of being defined and delimited. The author of Airs, Waters, Places, for example, begins his treatise, "Whoever wishes to pursue medicine correctly must proceed in the following way" (Aer. 1 = 2.12 L.).[49] The author of On the Sacred Disease, often thought to be the same author who wrote Airs, Waters, Places, wishes to prove the efficacy of medicine as opposed to the healing practiced by magicians, purifiers, charlatans, and quacks. These latter, he argues, say that the divine rather than the body itself is the cause of disease:

> It seems to me that it was people like today's magicians, purifiers, charlatans, and quacks who first made this disease [epilepsy] a "holy" one. It's just those sorts of people who claim to be especially holy and to know a lot. At a loss and having nothing to offer in the way of help, they alleged that the divine was the true cause of this disease and, so as not to appear completely ignorant, called it sacred. . . . But the cause of this illness is the brain, just as with the other major illnesses. (Morb.Sacr. 1, 3 = 6.354, 366 L.)[50]

And in On the Art, a work probably not by a doctor, although included in the Hippocratic corpus, the primary intent of the treatise is to provide an argument for the defense of medicine. "As to the practice of medicine, I will explain what it in fact is. First I will describe what I believe it to be" (De arte 3 = 6.4 L.).[51]

Authors of medical treatises specified in greater and unambiguous detail exactly where the parameters of their craft lay. There is widespread recognition within the Hippocratic corpus that medicine cannot cure all ailments: some ailments are inherently incurable (because either chronic or fatal), while others that might otherwise be cured have progressed too far for successful treatment. The author of Prognostic I asserts that it is impossible to restore every patient to health (Prog. 1 = 2.110 L.).[52] The author of Prorrhetic II, also considered an early treatise by some, proclaims that certain cases of gout are "incurable by human techne," at least as far as he knows (Prorrh. II 8 = 9.26 L.).[53] And the author of On the Sacred Disease alludes to the limits of medicine when he claims that epilepsy, or the "sacred disease" (ἱερὴ νοῦσος), is no less curable (ἰητόν) than any other disease, unless so much time has elapsed and the illness has become so entrenched that it is already stronger than the remedies applied (Morb.Sacr. 2 = 6.364 L.).[54] In other words, once an illness has progressed beyond a certain point, the procedures of a doctor are insufficient to conquer it.

Consequent upon the idea that iatrike is limited, the treatises assert the conviction that doctors need to recognize and abide by those limits; the good doctor should refuse to undertake both inherently incurable ailments and those brought to his attention too late. The treatise On the Art is specific and emphatic about these limits. Addressing the charge that doctors refuse to undertake dire cases, the author responds that such cases are beyond the power of medical practice:

> For if a man demands from a techne anything that does not belong to that techne, or from nature anything does not belong to nature, his ignorance is closer to madness than to lack of knowledge. For in cases where we have control due to our techne or to nature, there we can be craftsmen, but not otherwise. (De arte 8 = 6.12–14 L.).[55]

And later:

> [When people urge doctors to take on incurable cases], they are admired by those who are so-called doctors, but are laughed at by those who truly are doctors. For those experienced in this craft [of medicine] have no need of being blamed or praised so foolishly, but need praise only from those who have taken into account where the work of craftsmen has reached its limits and where it falls short. (De arte 8 = 6.14 L..)[56]

The idea that certain cases are beyond the limits of the techne is central to this entire treatise. At the opening of his discussion of medicine,[57] the author defines medicine by three elements only: elimination of the suffering of those who are ill, decrease in the violence of diseases, and realization that the practice of medicine is powerless in some cases (De arte 3 = 6.4–6 L.; emphasis added).[58] Only the true and good doctor, as opposed to pretenders and negligent doctors, both sees and abides by those limits, refusing treatment to anyone whose illness falls outside the capabilities of the techne. The author concludes the treatise by stating that not only his own words but especially the very deeds of doctors make clear that medicine has in itself well-equipped arguments for defense when refusing impossible-to-cure cases (De arte 14 = 6.26 L.).[59]

Other treatises present similar attitudes towards incurable cases.[60] Diseases II, which probably also contains material from the mid-fifth century, bluntly admonishes doctors, in certain occurrences of a wasting disease (φθίσις, which may be tuberculosis), "Do not treat this patient" (Morb. II 48 = 7.72 L.).[61] Similarly, Diseases I, which some date to the early fourth century BC, asserts that the doctor should treat to the very end those ailments that are capable of treatment, but in the case of untreatable illnesses he should know why they cannot be treated (*Morb.* I 6 = 6.150 L.).[62]

This attitude towards incurable cases is neither unanimous nor unambiguous in the Hippocratic corpus. Some works, like *On Joints* and *On the Diseases of Women II*, advocate treating incurable ailments (*Artic.* 63 = 4.268–274 L.; *Mul.* II 110 = 8.234 L.), while others distinguish between treatment meant to relieve suffering and treatment meant to influence the course of a disease. Most of the concessions to undertake untreatable cases are recommendations for supportive treatment only and are not intended to give the patient hope of recovery. And so *Diseases I* recommends giving what aid one can to untreatable patients even if the ailment itself is incurable (*Morb.* I 6 = 6.150–152 L.).[63]

It may seem odd to a modern audience that many of the conditions labeled incurable are not fatal conditions but chronic ones, such as a prolapsed uterus or epilepsy, as Heinrich von Staden has demonstrated. And so an incurable disease "grows old with" the sick person (συγκαταγηράσκειν) or "dies with" the individual (συναποθνῄσκειν)—that is, it persists until the individual dies but is not itself the cause of death.[64]

While among the Hippocratics there is thus no single attitude towards the treatment of incurable conditions, the refusal to treat such conditions is predominant. Such a stance was not a new one; Egyptian and Assyro-Babylonian texts contain prohibitions against treating incurable conditions.[65] What differentiates the Greek texts of the fifth century is the idea that the *techne*, not the practitioner, is limited. Egyptian tradition holds that the gods bestowed on men the healing craft complete and beyond improvement.[66] By contrast, the Greeks conceived of medicine as limited at the present time but as capable of expansion and improvement. The author of *On Ancient Medicine* describes this potential for discovery and development:

> Medicine has long had all things at its disposal, and a beginning and path has been found by which many excellent discoveries have been made over a long period of time. And all the rest will be discovered provided that the researcher proceeds competently, being aware of previous discoveries and using them as his starting point. (*VM* 2 = 1.572 L.)[67]

Thus, the good doctor chooses to abide by the present limits of his *techne* while realizing that those limits can be advanced.

The specification of the limits of medicine and the correlate refusal to treat certain ailments was crucial at this point in the development of the profession. In the absence of any formal method of validating the quality of healers, the true and good doctor had a social and economic interest in distancing himself from pretenders and unskilled practitioners (ἀγύρται and ἀλαζόνες) who might call themselves, or be called by others, doctors.[68] As noted above, the author of *On the Sacred Disease* distinguishes those who properly treat illness from magicians, purifiers, charlatans, and quacks (*Morb.Sacr.* 1=6.354 L.). The author of *On Ancient Medicine* likewise discerns a range of ability among doctors: "Some craftsmen are poor and others very good; this would not be so if medicine did not exist at all, nor would it be so had there never been any research or discoveries in the field, in which case all practitioners would be equally inexperienced and unlearned" (VM 1=1.570 L.).[69]

One very visible way for a doctor to prove his skill was to accept, and successfully treat, only patients with curable conditions. An uncured patient, after all, was not likely to attract future clients. As Jacques Jouanna puts it, the physician had to make two prognoses in rapid succession: one about the patient's condition and another about his own reputation.[70] While the treatises point to several reasons for refusing to treat patients with incurable ailments, including the possibility of harming the patient in the process of treatment, physician reputation stands out as a key factor. *On the Art*, for example, emphasizes reputation as the main reason for refusing certain cases. In an extended passage, some of which has been quoted above, the author argues that the good physician will be recognized as such by the right sort of people if he refuses treatment in instances where the ailment is beyond medicine's reach (*De arte* 8=6.12–14 L.).

Another factor that improved a physician's reputation was proper training. Since by definition *techne* implied more than common knowledge about a subject, proper training was essential for becoming a good doctor. Such training could not come from books alone but had to derive in part from study with an experienced doctor. In the *Phaedrus*, Socrates asks Phaedrus whether people would think that a man is a doctor who knows what to apply to the body to produce various effects like heat or cold but does not know to whom these techniques should be applied. Phaedrus replies: "I suppose they would say he's crazy, and that just because he had read some book or stumbled upon some drugs he thought he was a doctor, when really he knew nothing about the *techne*" (*Phdr.* 268b–c).[71]

The Hippocratic corpus emphasizes proper training repeatedly, even in treatises not considered to be advertisements for students or patients. The author of *On the Art* asserts that, "Effective doctors are those who have been educated not off-the-beaten-path (μὴ ἐκποδών), and whose natural ability is not horrible" (*De arte* 9 = 6.16 L.).[72] μὴ ἐκποδών seems to refer to training by a doctor or teacher recognized as someone skilled and qualified in the *techne*, as opposed to some fly-by-night operation or the relatively more widely accessible knowledge published in books.

Xenophon's *Memorabilia* vividly describes the importance of education to proving one's worth as a doctor.[73] Here Socrates parodies the speech of a highly unqualified candidate for the office of public doctor. This candidate, according to Socrates, declares that he has not studied medicine and has purposely avoided learning anything at all from doctors, even to the point of resisting the appearance of such knowledge. Socrates' sarcasm and emphasis on educational credentials demonstrates just how much education could matter to the reputation of a doctor.

The *Law*, a treatise of the fourth century BC or later, likewise addresses the issue of proper conditions necessary for producing good doctors:

> Medicine is the only *techne* in our cities that is penalized by nothing except dishonor. . . . Many men are doctors by reputation only, whereas very few really are doctors. Whoever is going to attain a true understanding of medicine must have the following: natural ability, a suitable place (τόπος εὐφυής), education beginning in childhood, love of toil, and time. . . . [The teaching of the *techne*] must be acquired with intelligence, and the education, beginning in childhood, must occur in a place well-suited to learning (τόπος εὐφυής). (*Law* 1-2 = 4.638–640 L.)[74]

τόπος εὐφυής is akin to μὴ ἐκποδών in *On the Art*, a phrase that stresses a right and a wrong kind of training, probably distinguished by the qualifications of the instructor, access to drugs and other supplies, and the like. The *Law* concludes with the admonition that only those who have been initiated into the secret rites of the profession can learn what is sacred (*Lex* 5 = 4.642 L.).[75] This admonition, couched in terms of a cult with initiatory rites, repeats the notion that the good doctor must undergo proper training.

Citing one's credentials, especially proper training, became critical with the gradual opening of the medical profession to those born outside families of doctors. In Homer, fathers taught sons to be doctors, as was the norm in antiquity where sons were expected to take up their father's trade. With the exception of mythic heroes like Asklepios and Achilles, who were trained to heal by the centaur Cheiron, no evidence challenges this model until the fifth century, when Hippocrates is said to have taught medicine to anyone who could pay (Pl. Prt. 311b–c).[76]

This opening of the medical profession to anyone who could afford to study fostered the growth of centers for medical thinking and teaching like those at Croton (the home of Democedes and Alcmaeon), Cyrene, Kos (where Hippocrates was born and spent part of his life), and Knidos. Misleadingly called "schools" in secondary literature, these were "at best . . . loose groups of practitioners associated with particular theories [and] teachers," as Vivian Nutton describes them, rather than formal, well-organized institutions.[77]

Nevertheless, after the field began to open to non–family members, medical training still closely followed a family model, in the form of apprenticeships served with a male family member, the local doctor, or someone farther away with a bigger reputation (like Hippocrates).[78] The metaphor of the family was maintained throughout antiquity in such documents as the *Oath*, in which one swore to treat one's teachers like one's parents. Such a measure to safeguard true knowledge, and thereby also the quality and standards of the profession, suggests a growing number of doctors, not all of whom were qualified to be doctors by proper training.[79]

Thus, by the late fifth century BC, with the proliferation of books about medicine and the opening of the profession to anyone who could afford to study, medical knowledge was not rigidly restricted. Anyone could claim to be a doctor and support this claim with some understanding of medicine.[80] But the good doctor attempted to protect his craft by recognizing and abiding by its limits, which meant, at times, turning away patients suffering incurable ailments. Those whom doctors refused to treat, or whose symptoms alone—but not the illness itself—doctors would treat, searched elsewhere for a cure.

CHAPTER TWO

Searching for a Cure

The Limits of Medicine and the Development of Asklepios' Cult

Healing is a matter of time (χρόνος), but sometimes it is also a matter of opportunity (καιρός).

Hippocrates, Precepts 1

It is logical to suppose that in antiquity, much as today, ailing individuals who consulted a doctor but were turned away did not just resign themselves to chronic suffering or wait to die from fatal ailments but sought help from other healers. The Hippocratic corpus itself leaves clues as to what its authors condoned as an alternative once the limits of medicine had been reached. While the medical treatises openly disparage certain healers, they never disparage the gods. Concurrent with this tacit approval of the gods as healers, the cult of Asklepios enjoyed a rapid surge in popularity.

Alternatives to Medicine: What Doctors Condoned

The author of *On the Sacred Disease*, as we have seen, minces no words about his contempt for most healers: they are quacks, charlatans, purifiers, and magicians, pretenders with no real ability to treat illness. Many of these same healers, he continues, mask their ignorance behind τὸ θεῖον (the divine), yet in so doing are in fact acting impiously:

They claim to know more, and yet they deceive men by proposing purifications (ἀγνεῖαι) and cleansings (καθάρσιαι) for them. Much of their argument rests on the divine (*to theion* and τὸ δαιμόνιον), yet it seems to me that their arguments derive not from piety (εὐσεβείη), as they think, but from impiety (ἀσεβείη) since they imply that the gods do not exist. I will demonstrate that their piety and their "*to theion*" is really impious and unholy. (*Morb.Sacr.* 1 = 6.358 L.)[1]

His demonstration of their impiety includes the following proof: when healers profess to be able to control the divine (by bringing down the moon, eclipsing the sun, or causing storms, sunshine, rain, drought, and other changes to the weather), they claim to be themselves ultimately more powerful than the divine (*Morb.Sacr.* 1 = 6.358–360 L.). Moreover, when they apply purifications (καθαρμοί) and incantations (ἐπαοιδοί) to the sick, they behave as if the sick were polluted by the gods. But a god, who is by nature completely holy, is more likely to purify and sanctify than to pollute (*Morb.Sacr.* 1 = 6.362–364 L.).

For this author, then, the claim that the gods personally cause any illness is inherently impious, as is the correlate assertion that any human can manipulate the gods into making them reverse an illness. Rather, "[t]he causes of disease are the same: the things that enter and leave the body, cold, sun, changing winds that never rest: these things are θεῖα (divine)" (*Morb.Sacr.* 18 = 6.394 L.).[2] "*Theia*" and "*to theion*" in *On the Sacred Disease* seem to signify the order to things in nature, which is itself divine.[3]

Thus, this author, as well as many other Hippocratic writers, believes that illness and health have to do with the divine inasmuch as factors like weather that affect the body are part of a divine order. The author of *Airs, Waters, Places* makes a similar claim in his discussion of impotence among the Scythians: "It seems to me as well that these diseases and all others are divine (*theia*), and none of them is more divine or more human than another, but all are alike and all are divine. Each of them has its own nature (φύσις), and none arises without nature" (*Aer.* 22 = 2.76–78 L.).[4]

The divine is integral to both authors' understanding of sickness and health, and their theory constituted a major departure from the model many Greeks used to explain illness.[5] To say, as these new authors do, that impersonal and indifferent divine forces infuse and control the world and have an impact on health is not the same as saying that the gods intentionally make you sick in retaliation for some deed and are thus personally responsible for your illness. This shift had a correspondingly significant impact on the model of healing: health is restored primarily through regulation of diet, environment, and the like, rather than through recourse to the gods.

This understanding does not, however, exclude the gods as a supplement to medicine in some instances. The author of *On the Sacred Disease* proclaims that there are occasions when visiting a sanctuary is warranted, such as when an individual has brought pollution upon himself. In this case, the healers "should have done the following instead" of performing purifications and incantations:

> they should have brought the sick to sanctuaries with sacrifice and prayer, in supplication to the gods. But people today do none of these things; rather, they purify the sick and hide the trappings of purification (τὰ τῶν καθαρμῶν) in the ground, or throw them into the sea, or carry them off to the mountains where they will not be touched or stepped upon. If the god was the cause of the illness, however, they ought to have taken these things to the sanctuaries (τὰ ἱερά) and offered them to the god. (Morb.Sacr. 1 = 6.362 L.)[6]

Although the gods do not pollute, they can help in eliminating pollution; hence, the need for prayer, sacrifices, and visits to the gods' sanctuaries. This author's acceptance of divine healing accords with the general piety evident in his condemnation of any healer who claims to have more power than the gods or who claims that the gods cause illness. "I maintain that a man's body is not defiled by a god inasmuch as man is utterly impure but a god is perfectly holy" (Morb.Sacr. 1 = 6.362 L.).[7]

Further treatises in the Hippocratic corpus indicate that other doctors were also pious and believed there to be room for piety in healing. The author of Book 4 of Regimen discusses the interpretation of dreams sent by the soul as an important tool of prognosis, and he advocates the use of prayer in certain cases where dreams indicate oncoming illness.[8] Depending upon whether one has received good or bad signs (σημεῖα) in dreams sent by the soul, one must take precautions and pray to the gods: "In the case of good signs, to Helios, heavenly Zeus, Zeus and Athena Protectors of the Home, Hermes and Apollo; if the signs are opposite, to deities that avert evil, as well as Ge and the heroes, that all difficulties may be averted" (Vict. IV 89 = 6.652 L.).[9] Later he writes that if someone should see the earth black or scorched in a dream, he or she should, in addition to other recommendations, pray to Ge, Hermes, and the heroes (Vict. IV 90 = 6.656–658 L.).[10] Prayer and the gods clearly have a place in this writer's methods of prognosis.

Elsewhere, however, the same author cautions against the use of prayer alone in healing. Early in Book 4, when discussing the role interpreters play in analyzing dreams sent by the gods, he mentions that these same interpreters also study dreams triggered by the soul (Vict. IV 87).[11] When they do so, they recommend only prayer, as in the case of divine dreams, because they do not understand how to counteract dream-signs otherwise: "Prayer is appropriate and entirely good," he writes, "but a man must call upon himself at the same time that he lays hold of the gods" (Vict. IV 87 = 6.642 L.).[12] As the rest of the treatise delineates, he means that diet, exercise, and other aspects of regimen must be altered, in addition to offering prayer, to bring about change. Health is not entirely up to the gods; humans must take responsibility and action as well.

The attitudes of the authors of early Hippocratic treatises towards matters of the divine and the gods can be summarized as follows: all illnesses are divine (theia) inasmuch as they have a nature (phusis) that can be identified and explained; the gods can play a role in maintaining health, and a person facing oncoming illness should therefore pray to the gods as part of their regimen to avert illness (Regimen 4); moreover, healing in sanctuaries is an option, one neither aggressively condoned nor in any way condemned (On the Sacred Disease).[13] There is no evidence from medical treatises or from any other ancient source that doctors ever categorically opposed healing in a sanctuary.[14]

The concept of the divine in the corpus of medical writings is not consistent, nor was there a universal stance on the interrelation between the gods and medical healing. Moreover, due to the sheer variety of beliefs concerning the gods, it is likely that there were some doctors who did not condone healing in sanctuaries. If the latter is true, however, it is significant that no evidence has survived to prove it, especially since the authors of medical treatises were so ready to castigate other forms of healing.[15] Any sentiment that did exist against such healing practices must have been too limited to survive or potentially too controversial to admit.

Despite arguments ex silentio and differing views about the divine in the medical treatises, the evidence points to the following scenario: some doctors, by making certain concessions to deities and prayer while disparaging most other forms of healing, suggested that ailments they themselves could not treat were perhaps best left to the gods, prayer, sacrifice, and healing in sanctuaries.[16] Healing gods thus became a likely next-resort for patients whom doctors turned away.

Healing Gods

Beginning at least as early as the Bronze Age, the Greeks worshipped deities for their power to heal. Anatomical votives from sites such as Cretan mountain peaks, for instance, suggest that some people were requesting or thanking the gods for healing, but which deities got the credit is uncertain.[17]

In the Homeric poems, we meet a host of gods who heal. Some of the healing seems utterly inexplicable, like that of Apollo, Athena, Leto, and Artemis. It is Apollo to whom sacrifices are made to lift the plague he himself started in the tenth year of the Trojan War (Il. 1.43–67), and Athena, Leto, and Artemis join Apollo in using their divine presence and touch to heal the wounds of their favorite human combatants (Il. 5.114–122; 5.445–448; 16.508–529). Moreover, the *Odyssey* mentions a man who is cured of an unspecified illness by the gods in general (θεοί); the method of treatment is unstated (Od. 5.394–398). Paieon, by contrast, uses medical procedures to heal wounds suffered by the gods on the battlefield and by Hades at the hands of Zeus (Il. 5.395–402, 899–904).

In Greek literature over time and across genres, most of the gods, especially the canonical twelve of the Olympian pantheon, act as healers.[18] That many of the gods could cure illness accords with the fact that already in Homer many could also inflict it: Apollo sends the plague at the opening of the *Iliad*, Zeus causes illness among men (Od. 9.407–411) as do unnamed cruel gods (Od. 5.396), and Artemis can slay any woman she wishes (Il. 21.483–484).

During the Archaic period, material evidence also points to the worship of certain deities for their capacity to heal. Metal anatomical votives dating to the late eighth and early seventh centuries have been found at the sanctuary of Artemis at Ephesus, and several dating to the Archaic or Classical periods have been found at the Artemis sanctuary at Lousoi in Arkadia. At the sanctuary of Hera on Samos, seventh-century bronze statuettes connected to the cult of the Babylonian healing goddess Gula of Isin suggest a healing function for this cult of Hera.[19]

In addition to the host of Olympian gods who acted as healers, lesser gods and heroes also healed; many had associations with specific communities.[20] For example, Herakles received the epithet Ἀλεξίκακος and in one tradition was said to have averted the great plague from Athens in the fifth century (Schol. ad Ar. Ran. 501). Pan, too, was credited with averting plague at Troezen in the Peloponnese (Paus. 2.32.6). And Amphiaraos, one of the Argive Seven against Thebes and later a Theban oracular deity, was by 414 BC also a healer, as indicated by fragments of Aristophanes' *Amphiaraos*.[21]

All of these and more were considered healers by the fifth century. Individuals looking to the gods for cures thus had many choices, yet the popularity of the cult of Asklepios suggests that it was to him, rather than to other healing deities, that many people turned.

The Early Development of Asklepios' Cult

The early history of Asklepios' cult remains obscure, but both archaeological and literary evidence points to its expansion beginning in the fifth century BC. The earliest material evidence for the cult comes from a sanctuary about six miles inland from the ancient city of Epidauros. Here Asklepios was incorporated into a preexisting cult of Apollo, who had been worshipped as Maleatas on Mt. Kynortion overlooking what would later be the sanctuary of Asklepios.[22] By the sixth century BC Apollo received another epithet, Pythaeus, and a new sanctuary below Mt. Kynortion. This sanctuary became one of the most popular centers of Asklepios in antiquity.

Early remains of the sanctuary date to the sixth century and include several bronze vessels of ca. 500 BC, one of which is inscribed with the name Apollo Pythias and another of which is inscribed with a dedication to Asklepios by a certain Mikylos.[23] How much before 500 Asklepios or Apollo arrived at this sanctuary is unknown, but by the early fifth century literary evidence, too, points to the presence of Asklepios at Epidauros. Three of Pindar's odes mention athletic victories there (*Nemean* 3.84, *Nemean* 5.52, *Isthmian* 8.68).[24] These contests, which included boxing and the *pankration*, probably honored Asklepios, since no other games are attested from Epidauros.[25] Moreover, *Nemean* 3 names Asklepios (lines 53–55), suggesting that Asklepios can be linked with the games at Epidauros just as Herakles (lines 20–26) can be linked with the Nemean games mentioned later in the same poem (line 84). That these Epidaurian contests had garnered enough fame outside Epidauros by the early fifth century to attract athletes from Aegina (the home of all three athletes in the odes) suggests that the games had been around for some time.

Epidauros also was hosting panhellenic contests for music and poetry by the late fifth or early fourth centuries. Plato's *Ion* opens with an Athenian rhapsode named Ion who is traveling homeward from such a competition when he meets Socrates (*Ion* 530a).[26] Socrates claims to be unaware of Epidaurian contests for rhapsodes, which suggests their relative newness, although Socrates' (feigned?) ignorance is no certain proof of this.

While Asklepios' presence at Epidauros is secure by the beginning of the fifth century, it may not have been the god's earliest sanctuary. Strabo states that Asklepios' first sanctuary was at Trikka in Thessaly (Strabo 9.5.17 [C 437]). This accords with some mythological accounts that name Trikka, rather than Epidauros, as the birthplace of the god.[27] Archaeological evidence, however, is thus far inconclusive; no sixth-century remains of Asklepios' cult have yet been located at Trikka, although coins probably depicting Asklepios link him to Trikka by the fourth century BC and to neighboring Larissa by the fifth century.[28]

Asklepios had a presence also at Olympia by mid-fifth century BC. Pausanias saw statues at Olympia dedicated to Asklepios and Hygieia by a certain Mikythos of Rhegium (Paus. 5.1.26). This Mikythos, according to Pausanias, is the same Mikythos named by Herodotus as the slave of Anaxilas, tyrant of Rhegium (Hdt. 7.170). After Anaxilas' death, Mikythos retired to Tegea and later dedicated the offerings at Olympia in fulfillment of a vow made for the recovery of his sick son. The reference to Anaxilas dates the dedications to ca. 460 BC.[29] Whether there was a cult of Asklepios at Olympia remains uncertain, but the dedication demonstrates that Asklepios had been memorialized there as a divine healer.

The first datable cult of Asklepios outside of the Peloponnese is on the island of Aegina; Aristophanes' *Wasps*, produced in 422 BC, describes Bdelykleon taking his father, Philokleon, to a sanctuary of Asklepios on the island (*Vesp.* 121–123).[30] The cult also reached Athens in 420/19 BC, as detailed in an inscription celebrating its arrival there.[31]

Asklepios' cult may have reached still other places by the fifth century, although the evidence is uncertain. Corinth, like Epidauros, welcomed Asklepios into a preexisting sanctuary of Apollo, possibly by the late fifth century.[32] This sanctuary lies at the northern edge of the lower plateau between Acrocorinth and the sea and seems to have belonged to Apollo already in the middle of the sixth century. In one of several closed deposits, which archaeologists have dated by its contents to ca. 575–525 BC, was found the rim of a large mixing bowl inscribed with Apollo's name: Ἀπέ[λ]λονος ἰμί.[33] Vessels inscribed with Asklepios' name and a large number of terra-cotta body parts were recovered from other deposits spanning the last quarter of the fifth century to the last quarter of the fourth, but there is no way to determine exactly when the cult shifted its orientation from Apollo to Asklepios.[34]

At least three other sanctuaries of Asklepios, including Mantinea, Sikyon, and Kyllene, are usually dated to the fifth century, based on references made as many as six centuries later to individual works of art. At Mantinea and Sikyon, Pausanias saw statues by Alkamenes and Kalamis, respectively (Paus. 8.9.1, 2.10.2), and Strabo reports a cult statue at Kyllene by a certain Kolotes (Strabo 8.3.4 [C 337]).[35] While there are obvious dangers in dating a sanctuary based on mention of a single statue, the possibility of a fifth-century date cannot be discounted.

Even aside from these three sanctuaries, the evidence discussed above demonstrates that the cult had begun to expand by the fifth century to areas as diverse as Epidauros in the eastern Peloponnese and Olympia in the west, Aegina and Athens in central Greece, and Thessaly in the north (if Strabo is right about Trikka). With the possible addition of Sikyon, Mantinea, Kyllene, and Corinth to the list, Asklepios would appear to have enjoyed a relatively strong presence in the Peloponnese at this time.

The Popularity of Asklepios and His Healing

In the fourth century BC, the popularity of the cult burgeoned. According to some estimates, more than 200 new sanctuaries of Asklepios were established.[36] In the Peloponnese, where the cult was already thriving, it now also spread to places like Argos, Troezen, Halieis, and Gortys. Although the existence of Asklepios' cult at Corinth and Sikyon in the fifth century is questionable, it had certainly reached both places by the fourth.

Beyond the Peloponnese, the cult spread to Eleusis in Attica and to Delphi in Phocis.[37] Among the islands, it reached cities such as Eretria on Euboea and Lebena on Crete. The cult spread also to Greek colonies as distant as Balagrae, outside Cyrene in northern Africa, and Tarentum, in southern Italy. In Asia Minor the cult reached Erythrai and Kos in the fourth century and Pergamon by the early third. It entered Rome in the late 290s BC.[38]

In addition to the establishment of many new cults of Asklepios, certain sanctuaries that had been in existence were lavishly refurbished during the fourth century. These refurbishments occurred at Athens and Corinth, but Epidauros is the best example.[39] Ancient building accounts inscribed on stone and erected in the sanctuary record the construction of new buildings at Epidauros, including a small temple, a fountain house, a large theater, and an elaborate round building called a *thymele* whose function remains unknown; contemporary with these buildings was erected a long stoa, in which people may have slept while waiting to be cured by the god.[40] The building inscriptions record not only the amounts of money spent on the refurbishment but also the names and hometowns of its craftsmen, individuals and institutions that provided funding, and sources and quantities of construction materials, like marble and wood. The variety and quantities of these materials and skills, and the distances they traveled, indicate how major an undertaking this was.

Two other inscriptions from the mid-fourth century at Epidauros record the names of cities, from Thrace in northern Greece to Sicily and Italy in the western

Mediterranean, that received ambassadors (theorodokoi) collecting money for the Epidaurian sanctuary, probably to fund some of its building program.[41] The number and geographic range of the cities listed on even these inscriptions, which are fragmentary, point to the growing popularity and status of both the Epidauros sanctuary in particular and of Asklepios' cult generally.

As these new and newly refurbished sanctuaries expanded in size, number, and opulence, so too did the number of votives dedicated to Asklepios. At Corinth, deposits from the fifth and fourth centuries have yielded hundreds of anatomical votives as well as pottery inscribed with Asklepios' name.[42] Many sculpted reliefs dating to the fourth century and erected as dedications to Asklepios have been recovered from the Asklepieion in Athens, as have fourth-century inventory lists recording hundreds of votives of various types and materials, from silver cups to leather flasks and gilded knucklebones (probably of sheep or the like, used as gaming pieces).[43] At Epidauros, still other fourth-century inscriptions record more than seventy healing encounters with the god.[44] These sanctuaries bustled with visitors.

Evidence of Asklepios' cult also spread well beyond the bounds of individual sanctuaries via coins, votives, and other objects depicting the god (like the coins from Larissa and Trikka mentioned above), and via literary descriptions of the cult. Aristophanes' Ploutos of 388, for instance, describes how a couple of down-and-out fellows take Ploutos, the god of wealth, to a sanctuary of Asklepios to cure him of his blindness. Aristophanes' description of the sanctuary and its rituals is substantial, adding up to more than a hundred lines of the poem (Pl. 633–747).[45] Theophrastus in the Characters, published in 319 BC, characterizes a person of μικροφιλοτιμία, or petty pride, as one who fusses publicly over his bronze votive to Asklepios (Char. 21.10). And a prologue to an unidentified play probably by Menander compares newfound self-awareness to waking up in a temple of Asklepios (P.Didot 1.9–11).[46] Even Plautus' Curculio, based almost certainly on a Greek New Comedy original but produced in Rome, includes a scene set at the sanctuary of Asklepios at Epidauros (Curc. 216–273).[47] Although it is uncertain that any plays of Old Comedy had the title Asklepios, at least two of Middle Comedy do, one by Philetaerus and the other by Antiphanes. Since the effectiveness of comedy requires that its references be familiar to the audience, the appearance of Asklepios and his sanctuaries in plays of Aristophanes and Menander in Greece and of Plautus in Rome demonstrates the widespread visibility and recognition of the cult.[48]

References to the cult appear also in the dialogues of Plato, where both Socrates and Ion converse briefly about contests in honor of Asklepios at Epidauros

(Ion 530a), and Socrates appeals to his friends to offer a cock to Asklepios upon his death (Phd. 118a). Xenophon, in Book 3 of his Memorabilia, also relates a conversation between Socrates and his interlocutors in which they talk about a sanctuary of Asklepios (Mem. 3.13.3). The Athenian orator Aeschines mentions civic sacrifice to Asklepios in a speech of the late fourth century (Against Ctesiphon 66–67), and Aristotle in the Republic of the Athenians likewise mentions processions in honor of the god (Rep. 56.4). An early third-century epigram of Theocritus celebrates a statue of Asklepios before which its dedicant Nicias makes daily sacrifices (Ep. 8), and Herodas' fourth miniamb paints a vivid picture of two women who visit an Asklepieion that is teeming with remarkable works of art.

While many of these literary sources are Attic, by the late fourth century non-Attic sources, too, reflect the spread of the cult. Theocritus was a native of southern Italy who lived also on Kos and at Alexandria, and presumably had audiences in many parts of the Greek world, and Plautus wrote for a Roman audience. This accords with the trend suggested by the archaeological evidence: the cult had a fairly limited existence early in the fifth century, but by the last quarter of the fifth, and continuing through the fourth and into the third, the cult quickly spread to numerous cities across the Greek world and beyond. Moreover, the rebuilding and enlargement of the god's sanctuaries and the number and wealth of votives to him affirm the popularity of Asklepios by the fourth century.

Central to the development and popularity of Asklepios' cult is healing. Since the mythology of Asklepios from Homer onward focuses on his ability to heal, it is likely that healing played a role in the earliest of the god's cults. But again the archaeological evidence is inconclusive. The earliest cult-related evidence directly suggestive of healing comes from the mid-fifth century BC. According to Pausanias, when Mikythos of Rhegium erected a statue of Asklepios at Olympia in ca. 460 BC, he did so in partial fulfillment of a vow made for the recovery of his ailing child (Paus. 5.26). Yet Mikythos fulfilled his vow by erecting a statue not only of Asklepios, but also of other deities, including Zeus, Poseidon, Ganymede, and Amphitrite. Just how much of the credit for his son's recovery Mikythos ascribed to Asklepios is uncertain.[49]

By 422 BC, people visited sanctuaries of Asklepios particularly for healing. In Aristophanes' Wasps of that year, Bdelykleon sails his father from Athens to Aegina in the hope of curing his insatiable love of jury service (φιληλιαστής, Vesp. 88). This visit caps a list of unsuccessful and progressively more drastic attempted cures, including ritual bathing, purification, and Korybantic rites

(*Vesp.* 112–135). One of Bdelykleon's slaves reports, "When these other measures proved of no benefit, his son took him by boat to Aegina. There he put him to bed for the night in the sanctuary of Asklepios. But early the next morning his father was at the courtroom gate" (*Vesp.* 121–124). The implication seems to be that not even Asklepios could help him, so badly was the old man stricken.

Inscriptions recording healing events at Epidauros likewise attest to healing both as the primary function and the appeal of the cult at this time. These inscriptions, known as *iamata* and published on stelai erected for public perusal during the great fourth-century rebuilding of the Epidaurian sanctuary, narrate healing events that took place at the sanctuary as early as the fifth century (IG IV² 1 121–124).[50] Many begin with the name of the cured individual and his or her hometown. In the earliest *iamata* these hometowns include Pellene, Athens, and Thessaly, indicating that by the late fifth century people from various parts of Greece traveled to Epidauros especially for healing.

The inscriptions also include stories, rare though they be, describing Asklepios engaged in acts other than healing. For example, he puts a broken vessel back together and locates missing treasure, a lost oil bottle, and a lost child. He also punishes visitors who doubt the efficacy of his cures or who, upon being healed, fail to make the promised offering. It is remarkable that even in the case of the broken vessel, the adjective twice used to describe it in its reassembled state is ὑγιῆ, or healthy, a word related also to the name of Asklepios' consort Hygieia.[51]

The stele listing the earliest *iamata* bears the title "Healings by Apollo and Asklepios."[52] How much credit Asklepios, as opposed to Apollo, got for these cures is uncertain, but Asklepios is named specifically in the narrative of at least one of the early cures, whereas Apollo is named in none. Of the earliest healing experiences recorded on the stelai, eight of the ten describe the healer simply as "the god" (ὁ θεός), leaving his identification ambiguous. One narrative does not mention a god at all; the tenth refers to Asklepios. It is likewise difficult to judge from the nature of the cures which god did the healing. On Stele B, thought to postdate Stele A, a greater percentage of the cures are described in terms of medical procedures. Since Asklepios was a doctor but, according to mythological tradition, Apollo was not, this suggests that Apollo's role in the cures declined over time.[53] By the early fourth century BC, Asklepios' name appears eight times in the narratives, Apollo's never, which suggests that by this time Asklepios was getting a larger share of the attention and credit for healing.[54] The list of cities from which people came to visit Asklepios had also expanded by the early fourth century to include Aegina, Argos, Epeiros, Halieis, Herakleia, Hermione, Kaphyiai, Keos, Chios, Kirrha, Knidos, Lampsakos, Messene, Mytilene, Pherai, Sparta, Thasos, Thebes, Torone, and Troezen.[55]

Even sanctuaries of Asklepios that were not panhellenic drew local people in search of cures. Sara Aleshire's prosopographic study of participants in the sanctuary on the south slope of the Athenian Acropolis, for instance, indicates that it was predominantly local in character but thrived nonetheless.[56]

The evidence for Asklepios' cult thus points to a pattern of late emergence, relative to his appearance in the *Iliad*, followed by rapid expansion less than a century later. The concurrence of developments in the cult and in medicine is striking: just as medicine was delimiting and defining itself in the fifth century BC, early evidence for the cult appears. And in the late fifth century and the fourth century, as Hippocratic treatises continued to emphasize the limits of medical practice, Asklepios' cult rapidly became one of the most popular healing cults in all of antiquity, spreading to numerous places both within and outside of Greece.

CHAPTER THREE

Asklepios and His Colleagues

Doctors and Divine Healers

> Our ancestor Asklepios established our *techne* when he had
> learned to impose love and harmony on opposites, as these poets
> of ours say and as I myself believe.
>
> Eryximachos (fifth-century Athenian physician)
Plato, Symposium 186e

A Greek farmer of the fifth century BC has been suffering from a throbbing pain in his foot that will not go away. The pain has become so acute that he finds it difficult to walk at all. As a farmer, he depends on his feet for his livelihood—for all the labor involved in plowing the fields and harvesting crops and even in transporting his produce to the agora several kilometers away where it can be sold. He realizes that unless he gets help, not only will his foot continue to ache, but his family will soon be without food because he will no longer be able to work. At some point he decides to seek treatment from a doctor, but the doctor shakes his head and says that although he knows what is wrong with the foot—it's a difficult case of gout—there is nothing he can do to help. As the doctor gathers up his medicine box to leave, the farmer notices the image of Asklepios carved on its lid, the patron god of all physicians. "Perhaps a trip to Asklepios' sanctuary will help," he thinks. "Maybe the doctor-god Asklepios can heal my foot." (For an example of such a medicine box, see Fig. 3.1.)

Such a scenario is artificial; there is no evidence for just such a series of events, nor would all individuals have sought the help of a doctor prior to visiting Asklepios. Some might have sought help from other healers first, while still others would go directly to Asklepios (though the costs of travel to Asklepieia and of the various rituals incumbent upon those who incubated

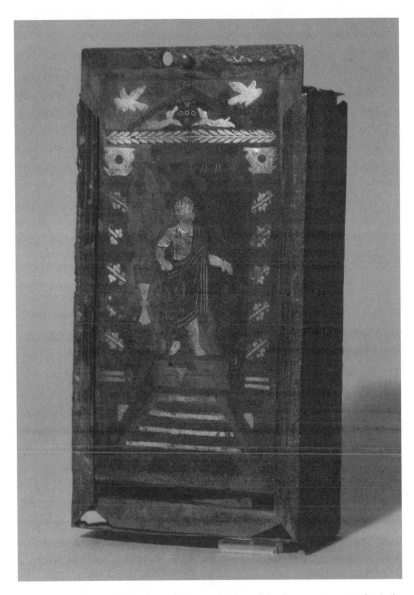

Figure 3.1. A wooden medicine box with metal inlay of the first century AD depicting Asklepios standing inside a small temple. (Antikensammlung, Staatliche Museen zu Berlin. Photo from Bildarchiv Preussischer Kulturbesitz / Art Resource, NY.)

there probably made this option a second or third resort for most people). Yet the rapid growth in Asklepios' cult beginning in the fifth century BC seems to have had a direct relation to the turning away by doctors of patients with apparently untreatable conditions. Those whom doctors could not treat were likely to seek help from the gods, given the respect shown towards gods and the acknowledgment of the divine by doctors themselves. The gods were not alike in their methods and credentials for healing, however. Only one god had medical training, directed all his efforts towards healing, and used many of the same techniques as mortal physicians. That god was Asklepios.[1]

Asklepios as Doctor in Myth and Cult

The mythology of Asklepios begins with Homer and is remarkably uncomplicated as to his function: he is a healer. Homer, as we have seen, portrays Asklepios and his sons as doctors (Il. 2.731–732, 4.193–194, 11.833) and indicates that Asklepios had to learn his trade: Cheiron guided Asklepios (Il. 4.218–219) much as Asklepios seems to have trained his own sons. In the *Iliad*, there is no hint yet of any divinity about Asklepios. Thus, in at least this one line of the early mythic tradition, Asklepios appears to be merely a mortal doctor.

The earliest source to identify Asklepios as Apollo's son is Hesiod (MW fr. 51), and most accounts thereafter in antiquity would maintain this lineage.[2] But Asklepios never loses his identity as a doctor, nor does having a divine father, even one known for healing, exempt him from having to learn his trade.[3] Moreover, as with any doctor, there are limits on how far Asklepios may go to heal. Already in Hesiod, Asklepios is punished with death for raising someone from the dead (MW fr. 51). Later tradition generally holds that Zeus grew angry at Asklepios upon learning of this transgression and hurled him into Hades with a flash of his lightning bolt, which in turn prompted Asklepios' father, Apollo, to kill the Cyclopes, Zeus' thunderboltmakers. Never one to be outdone by his children, Zeus retaliated by making Apollo serve the mortal Admetus for one year. Although Zeus would eventually bring Asklepios back from Hades and make him immortal, Asklepios would never again restore anyone to life.[4]

It is no surprise that this very act of raising someone from the dead—and thus overstepping his proper bounds, an inherently hubristic act—remains the focus of Asklepios' myth in fifth-century tragedy and epinician (e.g., Aesch. *Ag.* 1022–1024; Eur. *Alc.* 1–7), the only frequent variable being whom he brings back to life.[5] Pindar uses this myth as the centerpiece of his third Pythian ode, addressed to Hieron, ruler of Syracuse. Unlike most of the Pythian odes, which celebrate athletic victories, the occasion of this ode is an unnamed illness Hieron happens to be suffering at the time; thus the myth of Asklepios makes sense in this context. Moreover, as we shall see, Pindar focuses in detail on the transgressions and punishment of both Asklepios and his mother, and so the myth serves as a typical Pindaric tale about the dangers of hubris (and, in this case, of avarice—fitting for a cautionary tale addressed to a wealthy potentate). Since this ode contains one of the most detailed accounts of Asklepios, I quote part of it here.

After telling the story of the union of Apollo and Koronis, by which Asklepios is conceived, Pindar tells of Koronis' affair with a stranger. Apollo, angered at Koronis' betrayal, has his sister send a deadly plague upon her, but resolves to save his unborn son from Koronis' funeral pyre.

> But when her relatives had placed the girl   38
> within the pyre's wooden wall and the fierce blaze
> of Hephaistos ran around it, then Apollo said: "No longer   40
> shall I endure in my soul to destroy my own offspring
> by a most pitiful death along with his mother's heavy
>   suffering."
> Thus he spoke, and with his first stride came
>   and snatched the child
> from the corpse, while the burning flame parted for him.
> He took him and gave him to the Magnesian Centaur   45
> for instruction in healing the diseases that plague men
>   (καί ῥά νιν Μάγνητι φέρων πόρε Κενταύρῳ διδάξαι
>   πολυπήμονας ἀνθρώποισιν ἰᾶσθαι νόσους).[6]
>
> Now all who came to him afflicted with natural sores
> or with limbs wounded by gray bronze
> or by far-flung stone,
> or with bodies wracked by summer fever   50
>   or winter chill, he relieved of their various ills and
> restored them; some he tended with calming
>   incantations (μαλακαῖς ἐπαοιδαῖς),
> while others drank soothing potions (προσανέα),
>   or he applied remedies (φάρμακα) to all parts
> of their bodies; still others he raised up with surgery (τομαῖς).

But even wisdom is enthralled to gain.
Gold appearing in his hands   55
    with its lordly wage
prompted even him to bring back from death a man
already carried off. But then, with a cast from his hands,
    Kronos' son took the breath from both men's breasts
in an instant; the flash of lightning hurled down doom.
It is necessary to seek what is proper from the gods
    with our mortal minds,
by knowing what lies at our feet and what kind of destiny   60
    is ours. . . .

            (*Pyth.* 3.38–60; trans. William H. Race in Race 1997)

Pythian 3 characterizes Asklepios in much the same way Homer describes him. He is a doctor (63–67) and craftsman of his trade (τέκτων, 6) and must undergo training with the centaur Cheiron to achieve this status (45–46). But Asklepios also faces certain limitations. These limitations, like those faced by all good doctors, are external to the healer rather than inherent (imposed by the sovereignty of Zeus in the case of the former, and by the limits of the *techne* in the latter).

Most of the healing techniques attributed to Asklepios in this ode also resemble those employed by Homeric doctors and described in the Hippocratic corpus: Asklepios applies drugs, either externally in the form of poultices or internally via potions, and he performs surgery (51–53). In the same poem Asklepios uses incantations (*epaoidoi*, 51), a technique rarely associated with doctors.[7] His use of incantations makes sense inasmuch as supernatural methods are consistent with his divine lineage. One effect of these affinities and distinctions between Asklepios and other doctors in Pindar and evident throughout much of the mythic tradition is to characterize Asklepios as a doctor while simultaneously elevating him above his mortal counterparts. As a super-doctor of sorts, Asklepios is capable of more than any human physician—even to the point of raising the dead (even though this power is curtailed by Zeus).

Affinities between doctors and Asklepios apparent in the mythic tradition are evident also in cult practice by the late fifth century BC.[8] The earliest of the Epidaurian *iamata* mention instances of the application of drugs to the eyes, surgical removal and reattachment of parts of the body, the cutting open and sewing up of the belly, removal of material from the belly after it has been cut open, and the draining of fluid from the body.[9] Here is how the *iamata* describe the last procedure:

Arata of Laconia, hydrops. Her mother slept here on behalf of her daughter who remained in Lacedaimon, and she sees a dream. It seemed that the god cut off her daughter's head and hung her body with the neck towards the ground. When a lot of fluid had run out, he untied her body and put her head back on her neck. After she saw this dream, she returned to Lacedaimon and found that her daughter was healthy and had seen the same dream. (IG IV² 1 122.1–6 = LiDonnici 1995 [B1])[10]

Hippocratic humoral theory almost certainly influenced this method of treatment. According to humoral theory, the body contains certain fundamental fluids, or humors, such as bile, blood, and phlegm.[11] In a healthy body these humors are in balance with one another; illness results from an imbalance. Thus, to heal the body, one rebalances the humors by ridding the body of whatever humor is in excess. The draining of fluid from Arata's body would have restored humoral balance. While other healers may have had a similar view of the functioning of the body, it seems likely, given that Asklepios was himself a doctor and patron of physicians, that Hippocratic humoral theory exerted a direct influence on treatment at Asklepieia; his worshippers expected the god to behave like a physician. The cult thus appears to have accepted not just the mechanics of medical practice but also medicine's account of illness and health.

In other narratives from Epidauros, the god draws weapons out of the body (much as Asklepios' son Machaon does in the Iliad), grinds and pours drugs, excises growths, and administers emetics. All of these procedures are typical of doctors, even if the extent to which they are carried, such as the reattachment of limbs or the regeneration of an eyeball, seems superhuman.

Some iamata mention treatment by animals. Snakes and dogs most often, but also horses and geese, would lick or otherwise touch the afflicted area.[12] Here is the narrative of one such treatment, which takes place in a building called an abaton (perhaps the long stoa in which the iamata were recovered, although this is not certain):

A man's toe was healed by a snake. He was suffering terribly from a difficult wound on his toe, and during the day was carried outside by servants and was sitting on some seat. When sleep overtook him, a snake came out of the abaton and healed his toe with its tongue; after it had done this, it returned to the abaton. When the man awoke, he was healthy and said that he had seen a vision: a handsome young man seemed to have sprinkled a drug over his toe. (IG IV² 1 121.113–119 = LiDonnici 1995 [A17])[13]

The narrative provides a dual explanation, one that states what was happening to the man while he slept (a snake licked his toe) and the other that tells what the man dreamt had occurred (a youth applied drugs to his toe). Thus, even treatment by an animal, whether actual or imagined, could be conflated consciously or subconsciously with medical procedures. A good illustration of such a conflation, in this case also involving a snake, appears on a relief dedicated to another healing god, Amphiaraos (Fig. 3.2), whose cult will be discussed in more detail below. The snake seems to lick or bite the worshipper's shoulder while the god applies an instrument—perhaps a scalpel—to the same area.[14]

The *iamata* are our richest source for Asklepios' cures, but even in the early period of the cult the description of his use of medical procedures was not limited to a single type of witness; works of comedy and history tell a similar story.

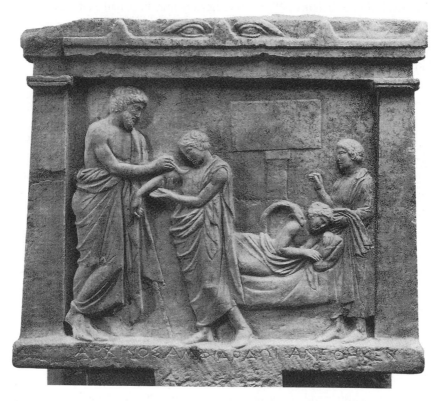

Figure 3.2. A marble relief from the early fourth century BC depicting the healing deity Amphiaraos treating a patient. The inscription reads: "Archinos erected this for Amphiaraos." (National Archaeological Museum, Athens, 3369. Photo reproduced by permission of the National Archaeological Museum, Athens.)

In the *Ploutos*, Asklepios carries a pestle, mortar, and medicine chest (κιβώτιον) as he makes the rounds among his ailing worshippers (Pl. 707–711), and he mixes various plants and spices to make a poultice for the eyes of a certain Neokleides (Pl. 715–723). Moreover, according to the fifth-century historian Hippys of Rhegium, a woman suffering from an intestinal worm visited an Asklepieion where temple attendants severed her head from her neck and drew out the worm, after which Asklepios reattached her head.[15] Here again, although severing the head from the body is hardly typical of medicine, surgery as a method of healing is, and Asklepios' divine abilities make such extreme surgery possible.

Nonliterary sources, too, confirm that Asklepios used medical techniques. For instance, the relief celebrating Asklepios' arrival in Athens, which will be discussed in Chapter 4, depicts the god next to a cupping instrument and forceps. Such tools are common on monuments of doctors, as discussed in Chapter 1 and pictured in Figures 1.1 and 1.3, but they are extremely rare in depictions of any deity other than Asklepios.[16] By the late fourth century BC, the city of Epidauros even minted coins with Asklepios on one side and a cupping instrument on the other.[17]

As time went by, Asklepios' cures shared a somewhat different affinity with practices of medicine. Inscriptions of the second century BC from Lebena on Crete detail cures that include careful lists of drugs to be assembled and administered by the patients themselves, similar to prescriptions given by doctors.[18] While at Epidauros only general terms like *pharmaka* or ποία (herb) describe a drug, the Lebena *iamata* mention specific plants like chestnut, myrtle, laurel, and lettuce. One even lists a cupping instrument (σικύα) as part of a cure.[19] In the second century AD, Aelius Aristides' *Sacred Tales*, which vividly recount his own healing experiences under the care of Asklepios, include bloodlettings and regimens for diet and exercise, as well as drugs and poultices. These increasingly descriptive narratives reflect a growing familiarity with medicine (or at least a general knowledge of how a medical prescription might sound) among those who incubated in Asklepios' sanctuaries.[20]

Since Asklepios is a god, it should come as no surprise that his healing in sanctuaries as in myth also included supernatural techniques. For instance, one of the early *iamata* from Epidauros states that the god made a woman pregnant simply by touching her with his hand.[21] In another instance, a mute boy who performs sacrifices and rituals in the sanctuary is suddenly able to speak.[22] These cures sound much like the kind Apollo performs in the *Iliad*, a healing by presence or mere touch. The *Ploutos* of Aristophanes likewise combines supernatural and medical techniques. Asklepios carries around a mortar, pestle, and medicine kit and mixes drugs for some incubants, but he heals Ploutos by putting a scarf over the blind god's head and beckoning sacred snakes to lick his eyes (Pl. 727–738).

Other Healing Gods and Heroes

While many gods shared with Asklepios the ability to heal, Asklepios differed from his immortal counterparts in several significant ways. Other gods who heal seem to have been born with the knowledge rather than needing to train to acquire it; they often function as much more than healers; and when they heal, they employ techniques unusual among doctors.[23]

Asklepios' father, Apollo, is a prime example of this type of divine healer. Known for his healing skills, Apollo was renowned also for his powers of prophecy, poetry, and even archery, as evident, for example, in the Homeric Hymn to Apollo. Nor is there any tradition that he ever had to learn to heal; his ability seems innate. Finally, in myth and cult, Apollo's methods of healing, as far as we know, do not involve surgery, bandages, poultices, or other techniques associated with doctors; rather, he heals most often in inexplicable ways. In the Iliad, for example, when Apollo heals Glaukos of an arrow wound, he does so in a manner described only as making the pains cease, staunching the blood, and putting strength into Glaukos' heart (Il. 16.527–531). Exactly how he accomplishes this is not stated. Later he is known for healing simply by raising his arm on high, which earns him the epithet Ὑπερδέξιος.[24] While Euripides in the Alkestis mentions drugs (φάρμακα) in relation to Apollo, there is no indication that the god uses them to heal; rather, he gives them to the descendants of Asklepios (Eur. Alc. 969).

Apollo did receive the epithet iatros, doctor, as attested in Asia Minor and the Black Sea region as early as the sixth century BC, although how or whether this epithet reflected a change in healing technique is uncertain.[25] In Greece itself Apollo seems not to have had a presence as a doctor until the late fifth century. One of the earliest literary references to Apollo's being a doctor occurs in Aristophanes' Birds (Av. 584), which was produced in Athens in 414 BC, that is, after Asklepios' arrival in that city and after his cult at Epidauros had reached panhellenic fame, and therefore Apollo's being so described may have resulted from these latter events.[26] Even Apollo's identity as a doctor in the Black Sea area seems in at least some cases to relate to his son's acts of healing: a fourth-century Athenian sculptor named Stratonides dedicated a statue to "Apollo iatros" in Olbia as well as one to Asklepios in Athens.[27]

Apollo may thus have acquired the "*iatros*" after his name (without undergoing any special training or change in technique) to enhance his appeal or even his authority at a time when interest in medicine and the cult of Asklepios was increasing.

Rarely do we glimpse any god other than Asklepios employing medical procedures on human patients. Paieon uses surgery and drugs in the *Iliad*, but he employs them to treat gods, not men. Moreover, he seems to have been assimilated into Apollo soon after Homer, hence the name Apollo Paian and Apollo's subsequent position as healer of the gods.[28] According to some ancient sources, Athena Hygieia, who had a sanctuary on the Acropolis, prescribed drugs to treat one of Pericles' workmen, but the sources are of Roman date and probably reflect the healing practices of Asklepios' cult at that time (Plin. NH 22.44, also Plut. *Per.* 13.12–13).[29] Asklepios is unique in being the only Greek god whom the surviving evidence for both myth and cult consistently represents as a deified doctor.

Asklepios' dual nature as a deified doctor is rare among healing heroes. In Attica, for which cults of healing heroes are better documented than elsewhere in Greece, prominent healing heroes of the Classical period include Amphiaraos (Ἀμφιάραος), Amynos (Ἄμυνος), and the anonymous Hero-Doctor, or Heros Iatros (Ἥρως ἰατρός).[30]

Amphiaraos, an Argive hero, was healing at his sanctuary in Oropos on the border of Boeotia and Attica by the late fifth century. Inscriptions and votive stelai of the fourth century indicate that Amphiaraos, like Asklepios, appeared to his worshippers in dreams and employed procedures such as surgery common to doctors.[31] The most famous and descriptive piece of evidence for the manner in which Amphiaraos cured is the votive relief from the early fourth century BC inscribed "Archinos erected this for Amphiaraos" (Ἀρχῖνος Ἀμφιαράωι ἀνέθηκεν) (Fig. 3.2, above). The relief has been interpreted as depicting three vignettes of Archinos' healing experience: to the left, Amphiaraos applies a scalpel to Archinos' shoulder (this presumably is what Archinos experienced in his dream); in the middle, Archinos is licked or bitten by a snake as he sleeps (what Archinos believes happened to him as he dreamed that Amphiaraos was treating his shoulder); and to the right, Archinos stands next to a depiction of the stele he is dedicating in thanks for being healed.[32] If this interpretation is correct, then Amphiaraos' cure, with its dual interpretation combining a dream of the god applying a medical technique alongside belief that an animal touched the affected area, closely resembles some of Asklepios' cures (especially IG IV² 1 121.113–119 = LiDonnici 1995 [A17], mentioned above).

Unlike Asklepios, however, Amphiaraos while alive was not a healer but a prophet. In myth, Amphiaraos was one of the original Seven against Thebes; as he fled the failed attack on Thebes, the earth swallowed him up at Zeus' instigation and the prophet became an oracle. Visitors incubated at his sanctuary in the early fifth century BC in order to receive prophecies.[33] Not until Aristophanes' *Amphiaraos* of 414 BC is there any evidence that Amphiaraos acted as a healer. Thereafter, Amphiaraos' function as a healer eclipsed his role as prophet and his cult spread to several places in Attica, but the myth of the living Amphiaraos appears never to have changed to accommodate his role as healer.[34]

Another healing hero, known as Heros Iatros, had sanctuaries in Athens, Marathon, Rhamnous, and Eleusis.[35] An inscription from Eleusis dated to the middle of the fifth century BC mentions this Heros Iatros in the context of a building contract, probably for the Telesterion in the sanctuary of Demeter (IG I³ 395; also IG I³ 393). His title, *iatros*, suggests that he was trained as a healer and employed techniques similar to those of human doctors, but almost nothing is known about him. Moreover, his cults at Athens, Marathon, and Rhamnous are unattested before the fourth century BC.

Also present in Athens was the healer known as Amynos, who occupied a sanctuary on the south slope of the Areopagus. Nothing is known of his mythology or healing practices. Although he occupied a sanctuary that itself may date to the sixth century BC, there is no conclusive evidence that any healer resided there before his arrival; the earliest evidence for Amynos dates to the fourth century BC. That he was a healer is attested by anatomical votives, some inscribed to him, found in the sanctuary.[36]

Among these Attic healers, then, only Amphiaraos and Asklepios certainly healed like doctors, while only Asklepios is known to have undergone training to become a healer, although Heros Iatros probably shared both of these characteristics with Asklepios. Given that the demand for Hippocratic medicine had increased by the middle of the fifth century BC, it may not be entirely coincidental that Asklepios and Heros Iatros were the subjects of cults by then while these other heroes probably were not, at least not as healers. As Asklepios' cult gained ascendancy, other cults adapted in order to compete. Amynos undoubtedly received some cachet from his association with Asklepios, who by the fourth century BC had joined Amynos in the latter's sanctuary on the south slope of the Areopagus.[37] The cult of Amphiaraos likewise attracted many worshippers after adopting medical methods. By the Roman period, Amphiaraos' son seems to have been identified with

Heros Iatros, perhaps another attempt to bolster the association of Amphiar-aos with medicine.[38]

The cult of Athena Hygieia on the Acropolis may also have been affected, but the evidence makes it difficult to interpret exactly how. The dominant read-ing of the evidence claims that the cult briefly fell out of favor after the arrival of Asklepios; another reading contends that her cult was established at about the same time or perhaps even subsequent to the arrival of Asklepios and his consort Hygieia. The former interpretation implies that Asklepios edged Ath-ena out in her role as healer, the latter that Athena assumed the guise of Hy-gieia in response to the arrival of Asklepios and Hygieia in their sanctuary on the south slope of the Acropolis.[39]

While many developments later in the fifth century, including the Pelopon-nesian War and the plague of the 420s, undoubtedly contributed to the prolif-eration of Attic healing cults, the exceptional appeal of Asklepios' medical healing was likely due to the fact that this divine doctor offered an attractive option for individuals unable to receive treatment from mortal physicians. The limits of the evidence make it difficult to determine whether the interactions of healing gods and heroes outside of Attica followed the pattern apparent within Attica at this time, but certain known factors would have promoted Asklepios' broad appeal in contrast to other healers. For instance, hero cults were often less mobile than those of other deities because their sanctuaries were traditionally identified with the place of the hero's death. By contrast, no one place could claim Asklepios as exclusively their own, inasmuch as Askle-pios' mythology is ambiguous and often even silent about the location of his death and burial. Even his place of birth was hotly contested in antiquity, a state of affairs that further freed him from local or even regional claim. More-over, Asklepios' profession implied itinerancy, as indicated by the walking staff commonly depicted in images of doctors and of Asklepios himself.[40] This itinerancy probably also enhanced his cult's mobility.

Asklepios' mythology was thus fluid enough in certain respects, like his place of birth and especially death, and fixed enough in others, like his profes-sion as a physician, to increase his exportability and widespread appeal rela-tive to other healing deities.

Doctors and Their Patron God

Further affinities between Asklepios and doctors fueled his popularity. By the late fifth century BC, doctors had claimed Asklepios as the divine patron of their profession. The doctor Eryximachos in Plato's *Symposium* declares, "Our ancestor Asklepios established our *techne* when he had learned to impose love and harmony on opposites [such as hot and cold, wet and dry, bitter and sweet], as these poets of ours say and as I myself believe" (*Symp.* 186e). By adding "these poets of ours" as another source for his claim, Eryximachos indicates that the idea of Asklepios as the founder of medicine was gaining wide acceptance and was of some age by the late fifth century.

In the Hippocratic *Oath*, which may date to the fifth century BC, doctors swear by Asklepios to behave properly towards their fellow doctors—that is, to behave as a member of a family or brotherhood claiming common descent from Asklepios.[41] An essential aspect of this familial metaphor was the claim that Asklepios was the ancestor of all doctors. The term Asklepiadae, or descendants of Asklepios, appears already in the fifth century BC, although scholars since antiquity have debated whether specific instances of the term refer to true blood-descendants of Asklepios or to all doctors.[42] By tracing their lineage back to Asklepios, doctors forged a powerful link between themselves and their divine counterpart. By doing so, they undoubtedly gained, and presumably intended to gain, authority and prestige among the population at large through this divine genealogy.

At the same time doctors touted Asklepios as their ancestor, Asklepios' cult forged its own ties to the medical profession. The *iamata* published at Epidauros, as we have seen, describe the god behaving like a physician. It is likely that the *iamata* contain some degree of interpretation and elaboration by the priests or other cult personnel who compiled the tales, and so it is remarkable that none of these functionaries expunged references to Asklepios' medical techniques.[43] The very least that can be said is that the cult personnel were unopposed to description of Asklepios' methods in terms of medical procedures; perhaps they even favored it. If it had been unprofitable to do so, presumably they would have amended or deleted such descriptions from the *iamata*.

Examples of the links between doctors and Asklepios later in antiquity give a sense of how the links forged in the fifth century multiplied with the passage of time. In the fourth century, for instance, doctors were dedicating votives at sanctuaries of Asklepios, sacrificing to him, and swearing oaths in his name. Inventory records from Asklepieia on the Athenian Acropolis and at the port of Piraeus list various medical instruments dedicated to the god, including cauterizing implements, probes, cupping instruments, small pots for the preparation of medicine, and physicians' writing tablets. While it is not certain that doctors made all these dedications, it seems unlikely that others would have had reason to do so, as Sara Aleshire has remarked in her careful study of the Athenian inventory lists.[44] Such instruments were also found in excavations of the sanctuary of Asklepios on Kos. In the Asklepios sanctuary in Athens, moreover, someone dedicated a statue of Polykritos, perhaps Polykritos of Mende, a famous doctor of the early fourth century BC.[45]

An inscription from Athens dating to the mid-third century BC mentions an ancestral custom in which public doctors sacrifice to Asklepios twice a year on behalf of themselves and those they have healed (IG II² 772.9–13).[46] That this is described as an ancestral custom (πάτριον) suggests that such sacrifices were taking place in the fourth century, if not earlier. In the third century, the poet Theocritus wrote an epigram about his friend Nicias of Miletos, a doctor who made daily sacrifice to Asklepios and who commissioned a wooden statue of the god (Epigr. 8).

By the first century BC, mythic traditions arose linking Asklepios and Hippocrates. According to a collection of letters falsely claiming to be by Hippocrates, known as the Pseudepigrapha, Hippocrates was a descendant of Asklepios on his father's side (Ep. 2, also Ep. 10, 17, 25) and dreamed that the god took him by the hand and gave him comfort when he needed assistance in healing a difficult case (Ep. 15). Strabo writes that Hippocrates derived some of his treatments from iamata posted at the Asklepieion on Kos (Strabo 14.2.19 [C 657], also 8.6.15 [C 374]). Likewise the antiquarian Varro, Strabo's contemporary, is quoted by Pliny as saying that Hippocrates had copied down cures from Koan healing inscriptions (NH 29.1) and that when the temple of Asklepios burned, Hippocrates established clinical (clinice, or bedside) medicine using these very cures (Plin. NH 29.4). Such influences were perceived as flowing also from Hippocrates to Asklepios. A mosaic of the second or third century AD that has been interpreted as depicting Hippocrates greeting Asklepios as he arrives by boat on Kos implies that Hippocrates and the medical profession had been established there before the arrival of Asklepios (Fig. 3.3). The bond between Hippocrates and Asklepios was advertised also on coins of Kos with the head of Hippocrates on one side and the staff and snake of Asklepios on the other. Hippocrates eventually received hero status and worship on Kos.[47]

While these legends about Hippocrates are largely apocryphal, by the Roman period other doctors were publicizing their close relationships to Asklepios. In the first century AD the Koan doctor C. Stertinius Xenophon, famous for his role as doctor to the emperor Claudius, made lavish dedications at the Asklepieion on Kos, including water supplies, a library, a naïskos to Asklepios, Hygieia, and Epione, and an altar to Asklepios. He even served as a priest in the

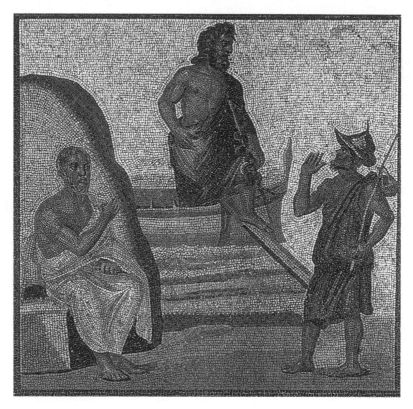

Figure 3.3. A mosaic from the second or third century AD depicting Asklepios arriving by boat, presumably at the island of Kos, as two men wait to receive him. The figure to the left is thought to be Hippocrates. (Archaeological Museum of Kos. Photo courtesy of the Ministry of Culture, 22nd Ephorate of Prehistorical and Classical Antiquities, Greece.)

cult, and coins were minted with his image on one side and the staff and serpent of Asklepios on the other, just as on coins depicting Hippocrates.[48] This Xenophon was not the only Koan doctor to publicize his ties to the god: two tombs of Imperial Roman date located near the sanctuary of Asklepios contain medical instruments and are perhaps the celebration of a more everlasting relationship of physicians with their patron god.[49] In Athens in the Roman period, doctors held the office of ζάκορος, or overseer of the daily functioning of the cult of Asklepios on the Acropolis. In Nysa a doctor dedicated a temenos and cult implements to Asklepios. At Smyrna the doctor Nikomedes, identifying himself as a servant (θεράπων) of Asklepios, donated a prominent statue to "Basileus Asklepios" for his frequent help in escaping sickness.[50]

Doctors themselves were thus in some cases directly responsible for the architectural expansion and general wealth of individual cults of Asklepios. And while such beneficence helped various Asklepieia, it no doubt also increased the visibility and reputation of the doctors who made these contributions. This may have been why Galen, doctor to Marcus Aurelius, repeatedly emphasized a close association with Asklepios. Galen wrote that not only was he a descendant of Asklepios but he had been personally healed by the god of an abscess (ἀπόστημα) and was advised by him in making at least one important decision while serving the emperor: Galen claimed that Asklepios told him in a dream not to accompany the emperor Marcus Aurelius on his German campaign (Lib. Prop. [Kühn 19.18–19]).[51]

While this dream may simply have been an acceptable way out of an unwelcome obligation, it nevertheless presented others with the impression of a close relationship between Galen and Asklepios, and it suggests to us that Galen knew he could benefit by creating such an impression. Furthermore, Galen claimed that Asklepios was largely responsible for his becoming a doctor. the god appeared to Galen's father in a dream and revealed that Galen would practice medicine.[52] Also, Galen was born, studied, and practiced medicine at Pergamon, home of one of the most popular and lavish Asklepieia of the time. He may even have held a position in the cult there.[53]

At the time Galen was writing his numerous tomes, the chronically ill orator Aelius Aristides was consulting Asklepios in addition to the gods Sarapis, Apollo, and Athena, and continued to seek help from physicians while under the care of the gods.[54] For Aristides, Asklepios' cult could function in tandem with medicine as well as other forms of divine healing.[55] Moreover, doctors participated in medical competitions held at the Asklepieion in Ephesus, and they toted images of Asklepios on their medical kits and rings, portable visual links between themselves and their divine patron. On one such ring Asklepios stands watching a doctor examine a patient (Fig. 3.4).[56]

All of this evidence indicates that as the cult of Asklepios continued to develop alongside medicine well into the Roman period, interaction between doctors and the cult remained strong. Had the cult at any point proven problematic for doctors, they would likely have severed all links with Asklepios; the converse is true as well. And so, beginning at least as early as the fifth century BC, doctors and Asklepios' cult enjoyed an active, amicable, and mutually advantageous contact.

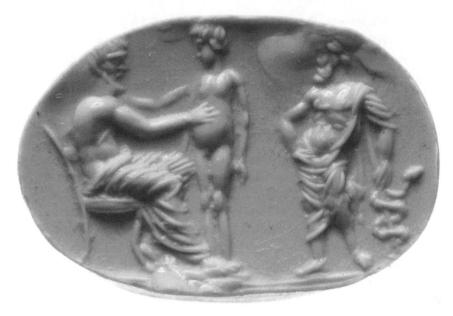

Figure 3.4. An impression made by a signet ring of the Roman period depicting a seated doctor examining a patient as Asklepios stands at the right watching. (British Museum, London, 1912.3–11.1. Photo © The Trustees of the British Museum.)

Asklepios' Specialization: Chronic Ailments

That Asklepios' popularity resulted in part from the reluctance of physicians to treat incurable ailments becomes even clearer when one considers the sorts of ailments Asklepios cured. Healing inscriptions from Epidauros point again and again to chronic ailments. For example: "Antikrates of Knidos, eyes. This man, hit by a spear through both his eyes in some battle, had become blind and was carrying the spearhead around with him lodged inside his face. While sleeping here he saw a vision. The god seemed to him to draw the weapon out and fit the so-called 'girls' (pupils) back into his eyelids. The next day he left healed" (IG IV² 1 122.63–68=LiDonnici 1995 [B12]).[57] Other reportedly cured ailments include infertility, paralysis, deafness, ulcers, tumors, festering sores, muteness, dropsy, baldness, φθίσις (a wasting condition of some sort), persistent headache accompanied by insomnia, stones in the penis, gout, stomach disorder, pus, worms in the belly, leeches in the chest, lice, and epilepsy. The overwhelming majority are recurrent or lingering conditions.[58] Blindness, paralysis, and infertility, moreover, appear among the earliest healing tales from Epidauros, as Lynn LiDonnici dates them.[59]

who practiced like a doctor but whose powers were farther-reaching—the deified doctor Asklepios stepped in to meet this very need.

The relationship between the cult of Asklepios and medicine was one principally of complement, not competition. Far from stealing patients from doctors, Asklepios treated patients that doctors found difficult or impossible to heal. Moreover, the god's use of medical techniques and his patronage of the medical profession speak of an interest on both sides of forging and maintaining mutual bonds that were obvious well beyond the medical community. While a complex set of factors was responsible for Asklepios' burgeoning popularity beginning in the fifth century, including the god's personal interaction with his worshippers, the ever-shifting political climate of Greece, and concern over health sparked by the prevalence of plague and other hard-to-treat illnesses, the medical profession itself generated substantial interest in the cult of this doctor-god.

CHAPTER FOUR

Documenting Asklepios' Arrival in Athens

Where a god passes, all around becomes hyper-charged with meaning: even the contingencies of his coming prove profoundly significant.

J. Z. Smith, Imagining Religion, 53–54

A sklepios arrived in Athens in 420 BC with considerable fanfare. Setting sail from his sanctuary at Epidauros in the Peloponnese, he docked at Zea harbor in Piraeus, where personnel from the cult of Eleusinian Demeter welcomed him warmly. A procession escorted the god to the center of Athens, and he was given temporary accommodation in the city Eleusinion, a sanctuary of Demeter at the northwest foot of the Acropolis near the Agora (Fig. 4.1). Soon after, Asklepios traveled by chariot up to the south slope of the Acropolis, where he settled in among notable neighbors: Dionysos Eleuthereus immediately next door to the east and Athena Polias just above on the summit of the newly refurbished Acropolis.

The arrival of Asklepios in Athens is remarkable for several reasons. First, it is one of the earliest known instances of the importation of the cult, as discussed in Chapter 2. Second, the event is unusually well documented. Little or no information remains about the establishment of most ancient Greek cults, and many assumptions about their early history are a matter of conjecture that began in antiquity. In the case of Asklepios, an inscribed monument probably of the late fifth century BC known as the Telemachos monument provides detailed information from a contemporary source.[1]

Third, the cult was given an especially choice location within the city. Few other cults introduced to Athens in the fifth century received prime real estate high on the slopes of the Acropolis, and still fewer were integrated into two of Athens' most popular panhellenic cults, those of Eleusinian Demeter and of Dionysos Eleuthereus.[2] Moreover, the cult of Asklepios itself quickly became popu-

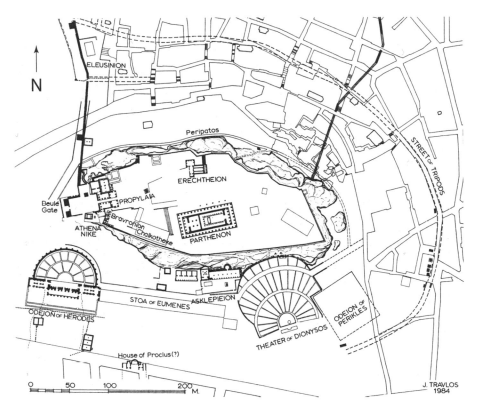

Figure 4.1. Plan of the Athenian Acropolis and surrounding area in the Roman period. The Asklepieion is immediately west of the Theater of Dionysos; the Eleusinion is northwest of the Acropolis. (Plan by John Travlos, reproduced by permission of the Archaeological Society at Athens.)

lar and just as rapidly had an effect on other healing cults in Attica. Votive reliefs as well as inventories from the Acropolis sanctuary document the high volume of visitors and dedications that Asklepios received from the time of his arrival.[3] And, as discussed in Chapter 3, other local cults, like that of Amphiaraos, that adopted healing methods akin to Asklepios' attracted strong followings.

Despite unusually secure evidence for Asklepios' arrival and the subsequent impact of his cult, no ancient source explains why Asklepios came to Athens. We can infer from broader trends explored in the previous chapters why Asklepios would have appealed to Athenians. Doctors were a growing presence in Athens in the late fifth century, as indicated by references to doctors in Athenian literature ranging from tragedy and comedy to the dialogues of Plato and Thucydides' history of the Peloponnesian War (particularly his account of the plague of the 420s) and by depictions of doctors on Attic vases like the Peytel aryballos and the marble disk found in Piraeus that celebrates Aineas, "best of physicians," discussed in Chapter 1.[4]

Moreover, as others have argued, some of the early medical treatises might well have been composed by Athenians. Although the manuscripts of the Hippocratic corpus come down to us in the Ionic dialect, this does not indicate that all the treatises were originally composed in Ionic Greek. Some of the early medical treatises, like On the Art, contain Atticisms that suggest Attic authorship and perhaps even an Attic audience. Nor would the treatises' strong sophistic element (no doubt the reason why some ancient sources credit the sophist Gorgias with having been Hippocrates' teacher) have been out of place in Athens at the time.[5] Furthermore, Plato's Symposium, an Athenian text, tells us that Asklepios was widely known at this time as the patron god of doctors. And one of the earliest iamata from Epidauros mentions that an Athenian woman was cured of blindness (IG IV^2 1 121.33–41=LiDonnici 1995 [A4]), a clear indication that Athenians visited Asklepios.

More-localized factors, too, undoubtedly increased Asklepios' appeal to Athenians, such as the plague that hit Athens in 430-426 BC. Any major threat to the population would have increased concern over health, and a plague as devastating as that described by Thucydides could only have exacerbated the desire for healthcare alternatives. Plague has dominated most modern explanations of the importation of Asklepios, but it is imperative to note that plague alone does not well account for the importation. I have argued this in more detail elsewhere, but the primary reasons are these.[6] First, the cult arrived six years after the last major outbreak of the plague. We must ask why the Athenians would have waited so long to import the cult if they thought it might in any way be efficacious against plague. Jon Mikalson has argued that Athens could not import the cult from Epidauros until the Peace of Nicias in 421 BC. Mikalson is almost certainly right on this point, but Athens could nevertheless have imported the cult earlier in the 420s from elsewhere, such as Aegina or Trikka in Thessaly (if Strabo is right that Trikka had the earliest sanctuary of Asklepios). Thessaly, moreover, was an ally of Athens throughout much of the war and, unlike Epidauros, would not have posed the difficulties incurred in importing a god from enemy territory.[7]

Second, and even more importantly, Asklepios is not generally known to have treated individuals suffering from plague. Plague appears in none of the iamata for Asklepios, nor in literary accounts, with two exceptions. Rome is said to have imported Asklepios from Epidauros in ca. 291 BC in response to a plague. However, the sources for the importation are late (the earliest being Livy, ca. 250 years after the importation) and may reflect a later tradition regarding the god's healing and/or the importation itself.[8] The second exception is in the *Sacred Tales*, where Aelius Aristides claims that Asklepios together with Athena cured him of plague in AD 165 (*Or.* 48.37–45). Aristides gives much more of the credit to Athena, however, whose rare appearance in the *Sacred Tales* suggests that Asklepios alone could not cure this affliction. The general silence in the sources about Asklepios' having treated plague is consistent with their silence about his ever treating fatal conditions; both seem to have fallen outside his purview, which makes sense inasmuch as plague is typically fatal. Apollo, Asklepios' father, was the great banisher (and bringer) of plague; he could lift miasma from an entire community.[9]

Third, it is worth noting that the only direct evidence for plague in Athens in the 420s BC is Thucydides' account of it. A. J. Woodman remarks, "Despite the impression created by Thucydides of an unprecedented and major disaster, the plague has (perhaps surprisingly) left no trace at all on any independent piece of evidence or inscription."[10] Woodman may be overstating the situation; in a forthcoming article, Carol Lawton argues that the plague did in fact leave its mark on the material record, in an increase in votives to gods like Asklepios, although this increase could also be explained by the war itself. Woodman is not arguing that there was no plague; rather, he suggests that Thucydides may have had rhetorical motives for describing the plague in such stark terms. In Homer, acts of hubris during war often result in physical debilitation for the community that commits them: a devastating plague attacks the Greek forces in the *Iliad* as a result of Agamemnon's impudent treatment of Apollo's priest. In much the same way, the severity of the plague in Thucydides' narrative may serve as a foil for Pericles' funeral oration vaunting Athenian accomplishments (Thucy. 2.34–47). In the very least, Woodman's analysis urges us to consider whether Thucydides' account of the plague is as objective and accurate as has long been accepted.[11]

While plague itself, regardless of its severity, does not well account for Asklepios' importation, the resultant general anxiety about health would surely have increased interest in healing gods, including Asklepios. So, too, did the dangers posed by the Peloponnesian War. Early *iamata* from Epidauros mention arrow and spear wounds, at least two of which were incurred in battle, possibly in this very war. Other *iamata* mention women trying to conceive, perhaps reflecting a larger concern about childbearing after the depletion of the population by war and plague.[12] Moreover, as others have argued, a mood of despondency followed the plague and years of warfare and may well have instilled in some the desire for a god who would give them individual attention.

Athens thus had abundant reason to import the Epidaurian god who by this time had earned a panhellenic reputation for the efficacy of his healing. Yet the Telemachos monument, as well as the location of Asklepios in Athenian topography and the festival calendar, suggests that these reasons alone are insufficient to explain his importation. Beginning with the Telemachos monument, this and the following two chapters will consider additional reasons why Athens had a markedly civic interest in importing Epidaurian Asklepios in 420 BC.

Sources

Scholars look to two main bodies of evidence to document the arrival of Asklepios: the Telemachos monument, which I will discuss below, and accounts of the life of Sophocles. The latter are late and problematic at best for recovering any information about Asklepios' entry into Athens.

Two accounts apparently link Sophocles with Asklepios' arrival. Plutarch states that Sophocles received Asklepios as a guest (ξενίζειν, Plu. Mor. 14.22 [1103b]). And the Etymologicum Magnum, a lexicon of the twelfth century AD, states that Sophocles received Asklepios into his oikia (house) and set up an altar to the god; for this reason Sophocles was called Dexion (Receiver) and was honored as a hero (Et.M., s.v. "Δεξίων"). Scholars have argued that these passages indicate that Sophocles housed or entertained Asklepios in his home upon the god's arrival in Athens. But, as Andrew Connolly has argued, both sources are vague as to the nature and occasion for these receptions and neither may have anything to do with welcoming Asklepios to Athens.[13]

Even granted the possibility that these "receptions" refer to an encounter between the poet and god on the occasion of the latter's arrival, both sources are late and draw upon material collected during the Hellenistic period when poets' biographies became a matter of erudite scholarship. Sophocles' vita is one such Hellenistic biography and, as Mary Lefkowitz cautions, these carry a large fictional element that can be difficult to distinguish from fact.[14] But Sophocles' vita states only that Sophocles was a priest of Ἅλων, Halon, a hero taught by Cheiron along with Asklepios. Halon is otherwise unknown, and Alfred Körte emended the vita to read Amynos.[15] Inscriptions dating to the fourth century BC from the sanctuary of Amynos south of the Areopagus do group the names Amynos, Asklepios, and Dexion, but Sophocles' name occurs nowhere in conjunction with them.[16] Nor does the vita of Sophocles mention his being honored as Dexion. The only certain link between Sophocles and Asklepios is a paean to Asklepios that survives in an inscription of the third century AD (SEG 28.225 = IG II^2 4510). According to a brief title on this inscription, the paean was written by Sophocles, but too little of the text remains to give much sense of its content, much less of whether the paean was composed for the arrival of Asklepios.[17]

There is thus scant evidence at best to support a tie between Sophocles and the arrival of Asklepios. Rather, it seems likely that the paean, and perhaps the proximity of the sanctuary of Asklepios to the theater of Dionysos on the Acropolis slope, generated a tradition sometime after Sophocles' death about his role in the god's arrival. The only secure evidence about the importation of Asklepios comes from the Telemachos monument.

Description, Text, and Translation of the Telemachos Monument

The Telemachos monument takes its name from the man whom the monument credits with establishing Asklepios' sanctuary on the south slope of the Acropolis. A T-shaped structure of Pentelic marble, it consists of an inscribed shaft chronicling the arrival of Asklepios and early events in the foundation of the sanctuary, surmounted by a rectangular plaque sculpted with reliefs apparently depicting participants, rituals, and architecture relating to the cult (Fig. 4.2). Luigi Beschi reconstructed the monument from marble fragments now in collections in Greece, Italy, and England; some of these fragments are ancient copies of the original.[18] The date traditionally given to the monument is ca. 400 BC based on letter forms, sculptural style, and a secure *terminus post quem* of 412/11 BC supplied by the last archon name (Kallias) to survive in the inscription. The party who commissioned the monument is unknown.[19]

The text and translation of the inscription are as follows. For lines 1–26, I follow largely the edition of Kevin Clinton (SEG 47.232), and for lines 30–44, that of Beschi (SEG 25.226), with minor changes as noted.[20]

[T]ηλέμαχος ἰδ[ρύσατο τὸ ἱ]-
[ερ]ὸν καὶ τὸν βω[μὸν τῶι 'Ασ]-
[σκλ]ηπιῶι πρῶτ[ος καὶ Ὑγι]-
[είαι], τοῖς 'Ασσ[κληπιάδαι]-
[ς καὶ τ]αῖς 'Ασσκ[ληπιō θυγ]-   5

[ατράσιν] κα[ὶ - - - - - - - -]

[- - - - - - - - - - - - - - - -]

[. . . . .] | | Σ[. . . .]Μ[. . .]

[. . . . . . . ἀ]νελθὼν Ζεόθ[ε]-

[ν Μυστηρί]οις τοῖς μεγά-   10

[λοις κατ]ήγετο ἐς τὸ Ἐλ-

[ευσίνιο]ν· καὶ οἴκοθεν

[μεταπεμ]ψάμενος δια[κ]-

[όνος ἤγ]αγεν δεῦρε ἐφ' ἅ-

[ρματος] Τηλέμαχο[ς] κα[τ]-   15

[ὰ χρησμ]ός· ἅμα ἦλθεν· Ὑγ-

[ίεια· καὶ] οὕτως ἱδρύθη

[τὸ ἱερὸ]ν τόδε ἅπαν ἐπὶ

[Ἀστυφί]λο ἄρχοντος Κυ-

[δαντίδ]ο· Ἀρχέας· ἐπὶ το-   20

[ύτο οἱ Κ]ήρυκες ἠμφεσβ-

[ήτον τὸ] χωρίο καὶ ἔνια

[ἐπεκώλ]υσαν ποῆσαι· Ἀν-

[τιφῶν . . . ἐπὶ το]ύτο εὐ-

[. . . . . . . · Εὔφημος·] ἐπὶ τ-   25

[ούτο . . . .]

[lacuna]

. ε.   30

ν ἔκτ[ισε καὶ . . . . . . κα]-

τεσκ[εύασε. Χαρίας· ἐπὶ]

τούτο τὸν [περίβολον ἀ]-

πὸ τὸ ξυλοπυ[λίο. Τείσα]-

νδρος· ἐπὶ το[ύτο ἐπεσκ]-   35

ευάσθη τὰ ξ[υλοπύλια κ]-

αὶ τὰ λοιπὰ [τῶν ἱερῶν π]-

ροσιδρύσατ[ο. Κλεόκρι]-

τος· ἐπὶ τού[το ἐφυτεύθ]-

η καὶ κατέστ[ησε κοσμή]-   40

σας τὸ τέμεν[ος ἅπαν τέ]-

λει τῶι ἑαυ[τὸ. Καλλίας

[Σκαμβωνίδης· ἐπὶ τούτ-

[ο - - - - - - - - - - - - - - - - -]²¹

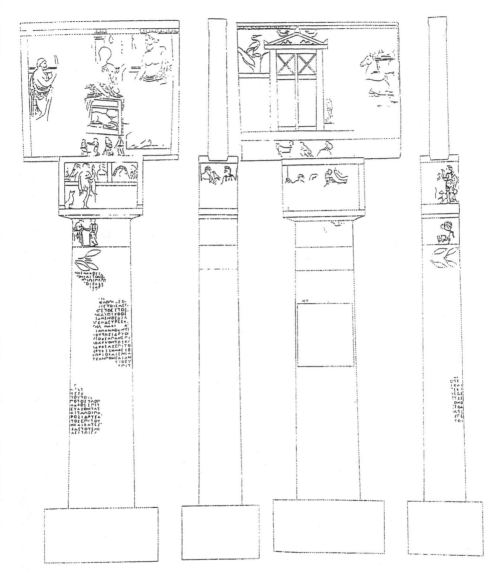

Figure 4.2. Drawing of the Telemachos monument, as reconstructed by Luigi Beschi, celebrating the arrival of Asklepios in Athens in 420/19 BC. (Drawing reproduced by permission of Luigi Beschi.)

Telemachos first set up the sanctuary and altar to Asklepios, and to Hygieia, and the Asklepiadae and the daughters of Asklepios . . .

Coming up from Zea at the time of the Greater Mysteries, he arrived at the Eleusinion; and Telemachos, having sent for temple attendants from the god's home [on the Acropolis], brought him here [to the Acropolis] on a chariot in accordance with oracles. Hygieia came along with him. And thus this whole sanctuary was established when Astyphilos of Kudantidai was archon [420/19 BC]. When Archeas was archon [419/18], the Kerykes disputed the land and hindered some actions. When Antiphon was archon [418/17] . . . [??] prospered. When Euphemos was archon [417/16] . . .

When Karias was archon [415/14], a peribolos was built apart from the wooden gateway. When Teisandros was archon [414/13], the wooden gateway was rebuilt and the rest of the sanctuary set up in addition. When Kleokritos was archon [413/12], the sanctuary was planted, and he arranged and adorned the whole sanctuary at his own expense. When Kallias of Skambonidae was archon [412/11] . . .

I have not followed Clinton in translating διάκονος as "servants" (lines 13–14) and οἴκοθεν as "at his own expense" (line 12). It is odd that οἴκοθεν should be used here to mean "at his own expense" while another phrase, τέλει τῶι ἑαυτὸ, is used later in the inscription to mean the same thing. As to διάκονος, according to LSJ it can mean servant, messenger, or temple attendant. Clinton argues that understanding διάκονος as temple attendants is not in keeping with the main purpose of the monument "which is to give due credit to Telemachos."[22] But it makes more sense, given the context, that Telemachos sent for attendants from Asklepios' new home on the Acropolis slope or from Epidauros (hence οἴκοθεν) to escort Asklepios here from the Eleusinion.

I have also not followed Clinton in translating ἅρμα as "wagon" (lines 14–15). LSJ gives no translation for this vehicle other than chariot. Clinton, who does not reject the restoration ἅ[ρματος], may have translated it as wagon since one other story of the importation of Asklepios mentions a wagon (to Halieis, IG IV² 1 122.69–82 = LiDonnici 1995 [B13], ἐπὶ τ[ᾶς ἀμ]άξας), and another implies one (to Sikyon, Paus. 2.10.3, ἐπὶ ζεύγους ἡμιόνων). I argue in Chapter 6 that the chariot has special meaning in relation to the cultic topography of the Acropolis.

Reading between the Lines

The fragmentary inscription on the Telemachos monument emphasizes Telemachos' role in the importation of Asklepios. His name appears twice (twice the number of any other human mentioned), once as the very first word of the inscription. Yet the monument is deceptive: as Kevin Clinton has remarked, the confusing mix of transitive and intransitive, active and passive verbs obscures the fact that the only credit Telemachos actually gets in the inscription is for moving Asklepios from the Eleusinion up to the south slope of the Acropolis (lines 12–16) and for setting up his sanctuary and altar there (lines 1–6)—nothing else.[23] Nowhere does it state that Telemachos brought Asklepios from Epidauros or even Zea to the Eleusinion, nor should it be assumed that one of the lost fragments credits Telemachos with importing the god singlehandedly.[24]

Telemachos' prominence in the account has led to the questionable assumption that nobody else, especially not the state, was involved in Asklepios' arrival.[25] But given that his involvement began, according to the phrasing of the surviving fragments, only at the Eleusinion, personnel from the Epidaurian cult almost certainly accompanied Asklepios to Piraeus, and personnel from the Eleusinian cult must have been responsible for housing him in the Eleusinion.

Scholars have suggested at best a very minimal role for the state in Asklepios' importation, but the state's role is much larger than anyone has heretofore argued.[26] Recognizing the state's role in the importation of Asklepios has been hampered by an attempt in scholarship to distinguish between public and private cults. Although the terms are often left undefined, it seems that what is most usually meant by "private cult" is that the cult was established or controlled by an individual or group rather than the state. Since most scholars consider Telemachos the primary or even sole party who engineered the importation of Asklepios, this cult is labeled "private."[27] As mentioned in the Introduction to this book, criticism has recently arisen as to the validity of the public-private distinction as applied to Greek cults. Suspending this distinction reveals that the Athenian state played an active role in importing Asklepios and establishing his sanctuary and cult in Athens.

Telemachos' starring role in the (fragmentary) inscription may be due to an ancient tradition whereby gods made their wishes known to a community through an individual, especially regarding the establishment of cults. Athena instructed Orestes to set up a cult in honor of Iphigeneia (Eur. IT 1446–1474), and Pan appeared to Pheidippides, on his run between Sparta and Marathon, to ask the Athenians to establish a cult of Pan (Hdt. 6.105–106).[28] Likewise, the founding of several cults or sanctuaries of Asklepios was attributed to individuals, as at Sikyon (Paus. 2.10.3), Titane (Paus. 2.11.5), Argos (Paus. 2.23.4), and Pergamon (Paus. 2.26.8). Thus, the mention of Telemachos may have more to do with maintaining a traditional topos than actual fact, although the two need not be mutually exclusive.[29]

Even if Telemachos did bring Asklepios to Athens all the way from Epidauros, such intense involvement by an individual would in no way preclude the polis from having been an active and even essential participant in the event. Although the precise role of the state in importing deities has been disputed, it is widely agreed that bringing a new god into Athens in the late fifth century would have required approval of the demos.[30] At whatever point Telemachos' involvement began, he would have needed authorization from the state to found the Acropolis sanctuary.[31] The Telemachos monument itself contains evidence of just such state interest and involvement.

The Eleusinian Cult of Demeter and Kore

Second only to the prominence of Telemachos in the chronicle of Asklepios' arrival is the cult of Eleusinian Demeter and Kore. The level of involvement of the Eleusis cult in the arrival of Asklepios, especially as documented in a fragmentary inscription of twenty-five short lines, is remarkable. According to the Telemachos monument, Asklepios came to Athens at the time of the Greater Mysteries in honor of Eleusinian Demeter (lines 10–11) and stopped at the city Eleusinion for an unspecified period of time (lines 11–12).[32] In 419/18 BC, after Asklepios took up residence on the south slope of the Acropolis, a dispute over his sanctuary there arose, at the instigation of the Kerykes (lines 20–23), a priestly family of the cult of Eleusinian Demeter who played a prominent role in the state as generals, ambassadors, and envoys. (One of their priests was reputed to have engineered the peace between Sparta and Artaxerxes and to have negotiated the Thirty Years' Peace with Sparta.[33]) The Eleusinian cult clearly had great influence on events surrounding Asklepios' arrival.

The Eleusinian cult also enjoyed strong support from the Athenian state. One of Athens' three major panhellenic cults (along with Athena Polias and Dionysos Eleuthereus), its primary festival, the Greater Mysteries, attracted visitors from all over the Greek world well into the Roman period.[34] The event was second only to the games at Olympia as the most famous of all Greek festivals. No later than the sixth century BC Athens had taken control of the Eleusinian cult, as attested by Athenian decrees regulating the worship of Demeter and Kore at Eleusis.[35] Athens' stamp on the cult is visible also in the introduction of Triptolemos to Demeter myth beginning in the sixth century.[36] According to the mythic tradition, Triptolemos was an Eleusinian who taught agriculture to humans after having learned it from Demeter; since the first earth he plowed lay near Athens, Athens therefore claimed to be the origin of agriculture.

In the fifth century, the Eleusis sanctuary continued to expand. Damaged by the Persian invasion of 480, it was rebuilt under Kimon and Pericles. While Persian destruction necessitated rebuilding, expansion of the sanctuary at the same time indicates growth within the cult.[37] Also indicative is the increase in size of the rebuilt Telesterion, the large enclosed building used for initiation rituals whose fifth-century footprint is nearly three times that of its sixth-century predecessor.[38] Its unusual form, a hypostyle hall, resembles the Odeion built in the sanctuary of Dionysos on the south slope of the Athenian Acropolis. The Telesterion and Odeion thus functioned as a visual link between Athens and Eleusis.

Further evidence of close ties between Athens and Eleusis is a sacred law from the mid-fifth century authorizing Athenians to use proceeds from the cult "as they wish" (IG I³ 6). As Maureen Cavanaugh comments regarding this law, "The close interaction of the Athenian state with the sanctuary of Demeter and Kore in this early period is striking."[39] In 405 BC, Aristophanes characterized his chorus of the Frogs, who essentially represent the Athenian demos, as initiates into the Greater Mysteries.[40] Such an equation points to the centrality of the Eleusinian cult to Athens and its absorption into Athenian polis-identity.

The rituals of the Greater Mysteries further publicized Athens' close ties to Eleusis. Those celebrating the Mysteries gathered first in Athens, which was the locus of at least half of the festival. At about the midpoint of the festival (scholars disagree as to its length, estimating about nine days beginning on 15 Boedromion), participants processed to Eleusis, an act that symbolically recreated a bond between the two cities and, according to François de Polignac's model of extraurban sanctuaries, articulated Athenian control over Eleusis.[41] By the fifth century BC, initiates had also to attend the Lesser Mysteries staged in Athens seven months prior to and in preparation for the Greater Mysteries.[42]

Asklepios' arrival in Athens during celebration of the Greater Mysteries cannot therefore have been without significance to the polis, especially given the many other rituals, surely not coincidental, that bound Asklepios solidly into the fabric of the Eleusinian cult. Not only did Asklepios arrive during the Mysteries, but a priestess of Eleusinian Demeter probably met him in Piraeus and escorted him to the Eleusinion.[43] Here the god resided for a time in the very place where sacred objects from Eleusis were deposited immediately before the start of the Mysteries and where sacrifices may have taken place during the festival.[44]

Moreover, according to Philostratos and Pausanias, an annual festival of Asklepios called the Epidauria was integrated into the Greater Mysteries, probably soon after Asklepios' arrival (Philostr. *VA* 4.17; Paus. 2.26.8). Both authors explain that Asklepios came to Athens to be initiated into the Mysteries, but because he arrived too late to take part in the preliminary rites on the first day of the festival, a day was added to accommodate him.[45] Asklepios' late arrival functioned as an *aition* for the day on which those who had joined the festival on time could rest, while those who missed the preliminary rites could now perform them. The integration of the Epidauria into the Mysteries, as with any addition or change to the civic calendar, required the demos' approval.[46] Little is known about the rituals of the Epidauria other than that they included a sacrifice, banquet, and all-night festival (παννυχίς), which are mentioned in IG II² 974 (second century BC). It is also likely that an annual procession from Piraeus to the center of Athens reenacted Asklepios' original route into the city.[47]

The ties between Asklepios and the Eleusinian cult articulated by the Telemachos monument and reinforced annually by processions, myths, and the festival calendar thus speak to a high level of cooperation between the two. The Athenian state clearly exerted great control over the Eleusinian cult and thus played a major role in orchestrating the ties between the cults of Asklepios and Eleusinian Demeter.

Even the land dispute vaguely mentioned on the Telemachos monument (lines 20–23) may be another sign of cooperation between the state and the cult of Asklepios.[48] The inscription states only that the Kerykes disputed the land and hindered some actions in 419/18 BC (οἱ Κήρυκες ἠμφεσβήτον τὸ χωρίο καὶ ἔνια ἐπεκώλυσαν ποῆσαι); the exact nature of the dispute remains unknown, including with whom and why the Kerykes were engaged in it, as does the specific time it took place within that year. If the Kerykes did oppose Asklepios' relocation to the Acropolis, we must imagine that this took place early in 419/18; otherwise, it becomes hard to explain why they would have waited a year or more to contest it. Moreover, the inscription clearly indicates that the

Kerykes successfully prevented someone from completing certain actions. This someone need not have been Telemachos. In fact, it seems odd that a monument that otherwise praises Telemachos' efforts would mention a dispute that he lost. Thus unless the Kerykes had sudden reason in 419/18 to want Asklepios off the Acropolis, it makes better sense to understand the dispute as involving another, unnamed party against whom the Kerykes were helping to safeguard the cult and sanctuary.[49]

The Location of Asklepios' Sanctuary

When Telemachos moved Asklepios from the Eleusinion, he brought the god not to an outlying region of the city or to an inconspicuous place near the city center; instead, he brought him up to the south slope of the Acropolis just under the brow of some of Athens' most prominent cults. Thucydides relates that the Acropolis was the oldest part of Athens and the site of some of its earliest sanctuaries.[50] In 420, the Acropolis was still under reconstruction in an effort to restore buildings destroyed by the Persians in 480; work continued on the temple and parapet of Athena Nike and on the Erechtheion.[51] And in the sanctuary of Dionysos, east of and immediately adjacent to what would become the precinct of Asklepios, a large music hall (the Odeion) had been built less than twenty years earlier, accompanied probably by changes to the theater.[52] The prominence and cultic significance of the Acropolis at this time implies that Telemachos must have secured the support and approval of the demos to build a sanctuary there.

The sheer size of Asklepios' sanctuary is also remarkable: it ultimately extended about 80 meters across the slope of the Acropolis. Although the dimensions of the original sanctuary remain uncertain, the possibility that Telemachos was able to acquire a strip of land as long as 80 meters on the Acropolis slopes further suggests that the demos ratified his endeavor.[53]

The sculpted reliefs crowning the Telemachos monument provide still more evidence of the state's approval. One of the reliefs depicts a large double doorway with a stork sitting in a tree next to it (see Fig. 4.2). Beschi has argued that these images represent the topography of the Asklepieion: the doorway is that of the sanctuary, and the stork, called a πελαργός in Greek, symbolizes the Pelargikon, or wall that surrounded the Acropolis.[54] If Beschi's interpretation is correct, this stork reflects the proximity of the Asklepieion to the Pelargikon.

An Athenian decree of the second half of the fifth century, IG I³ 78 (known as the First-Fruits decree because it regulates offerings of first fruits, or portions of the annual harvest, to Eleusinian Demeter), contains a rider that places certain restrictions upon activity within the Pelargikon (lines 47–61).[55] One such restriction prohibits the construction of altars there without the approval of the demos and boule (lines 54–59).[56] Since the path of the Pelargikon is uncertain, it is also uncertain whether any of the Asklepieion, including the altar built by Telemachos, fell within it. Yet the depiction of the *pelargos* on the Telemachos monument suggests that the sanctuary had a significant relationship to—and most likely inclusion within—the boundary. If so, Telemachos received the approval of the boule in addition to the demos to build the sanctuary where he did.[57]

The placement of Asklepios' sanctuary on land highly desirable, restricted, and regulated, combined with the careful orchestration of his arrival with the cult of Eleusinian Demeter, indicates more than tacit approval by the state. It indicates a major civic commitment to the importation of Asklepios.[58]

CHAPTER FIVE

Asklepios and the Topography of Athenian Cult

> It is somewhat remarkable that this intrusive cult [of Asklepios]
> managed to stake a claim within the feast days of two such cults
> as the Eleusinian Demeter and Dionysus Eleuthereus.
>
> H. W. Parke, Festivals of the Athenians, 135

Reading between the lines of the Telemachos monument, we find a strong civic commitment to establishing Asklepios successfully in the heart of Athens. The present chapter explores the nature of this commitment in greater detail by further investigating where the state situated Asklepios and his festivals within the topography and festival calendar of Athens upon his arrival.[1]

While certain practicalities played a role in determining these spatial and temporal loci (such as the presence of a water source on what became the eastern terrace of the Asklepieion), practicalities alone cannot account for the symbolic associations created by the loci.[2] In an area as symbolically charged as the Acropolis, especially in 420 BC, any alignments were capable of evoking meanings and associations that the state must have recognized and even invited when they made their decision about where to situate Asklepios.

Since it is impossible to consider all of the connections forged by the state with Asklepios, I will confine myself to three of the most visible: (1) the Acropolis and its slopes as the primary spatial context into which the sanctuary of Asklepios was integrated, and the cults of (2) Dionysos Eleuthereus and (3) Eleusinian Demeter as the cults with which the two annual festivals of Asklepios were coordinated and thus as the two cults having the most prominent ritual links to Asklepios.

The Acropolis and the Greater Panathenaia

When Asklepios took up residence on the south slope of the Acropolis in 420 BC, he was assimilated into the web of associations and meanings the Acropolis held at that time. It is common to speak of the fifth-century building program on the summit, initiated by Pericles, as a unity unto itself, even as a "text" whose meaning changed over time with each addition or alteration, and the structures on the slopes of the Acropolis must likewise have exerted their own influence and been influenced by those on the summit.[3] As Jeffrey Hurwit has argued, the themes of *agon* and *nike* prevalent on the summit were reflected in the dramatic contests that took place in the Theater of Dionysos, in the choregic dedications that flanked it, and in the Odeion built there probably to celebrate Athenian victory over the Persians.[4]

While a monument as prominent and culticly important as the Acropolis necessarily conveyed numerous meanings over time, one of the most constant of its identities was a locus of Athenian origins: here Athena vied with Poseidon over possession of Attica, and here, as fifth-century tradition maintained, the early inhabitants of Athens lived.[5] When the Athenians rebuilt the Acropolis under Pericles, they integrated these traditions into the monuments themselves. For example, the Parthenon's west pediment depicted Athena's victory over Poseidon. Moreover, a corner of the Propyleia was truncated to accommodate Cyclopean masonry of the Mycenaean period, and carefully positioned cutouts in the blocks of the Nike temple bastion provided windows onto the Mycenaean bastion below.[6] Thus, in 420 BC when Asklepios arrived, the Acropolis advertised its status as the oldest and most sacred civic space in Athens.

The monuments of the Acropolis also celebrated Greek victory over the Persians, who had set fire to it in 480 BC. Sculptural friezes adorning the Temple of Athena Nike and the balustrade crowning its parapet depicted Greeks fighting Persians—possibly the battle of Marathon itself. And as Hurwit has argued, even the battles between Amazons and Greeks and between the Olympian gods and the giants who threatened their power—depicted across the monuments of the Acropolis from the Parthenon metopes to the shield of the colossal statue of Athena Parthenos inside the Parthenon to the friezes and pediments of the Temple of Athena Nike—could all be read as allusions to Athenian victory against the Persians. So, too, could the dozens of sculpted, winged Nikes hovering over the summit.[7] These monuments assimilated recent accomplishments into the heroic age, thereby elevating them towards heroic status.

The defeat of the Persians in 479 BC led also to the creation of the Delian League. Its purpose, according to Thucydides, was to exact vengeance on Persia for the sufferings of the Greeks (Thucy. 1.96). This goal was apparently attained in the 460s when the Greeks defeated the Persians at Eurymedon. A formal declaration of peace between Greece and Persia may soon have followed (the so-called Peace of Kallias, whose historicity is disputed), yet the league continued and developed into an empire under Athenian control.[8]

By 454 BC, Athens moved the treasury of the Delian League from Delos to Athens, and presumably onto the Acropolis. This transfer openly acknowledged and further reinforced Athens' position, and it identified Athena as the deity of empire. Members now paid first fruits to Athena, income that helped finance construction of the Parthenon, her largest temple on the Acropolis.[9] The Parthenon housed offerings from Athens' colonies and allies, and inventory lists tallied its contents for public record (IG I³ 296–299, for 430–426 BC). Visitors to the Acropolis could also see posted on marble stelai records of tribute payment to the League by member states (IG I³ 259–272), as well as regulations governing its collection (IG I³ 68).[10] Even the *hellenotamiai* who administered the collection of tribute conducted their business on the Acropolis, and decrees concerning Athens' relations with specific colonies and allies (like Erythrai, Chalkis, Samos, and Brea) stood thick across the summit.[11]

In 420 BC the Acropolis thus became, among its many other meanings and associations, a monument celebrating Athenian empire. One did not have to be able to read the inscriptions to understand this subtext.[12] The images of Greeks fighting barbarians and the flock of Nikes concentrated on the Acropolis, for instance, all carried a potentially double meaning in the climate of the Peloponnesian War. At a lull that would last only until 419 BC, this war pitted Athens primarily against Sparta but also against many Greek states under Athenian rule. Inasmuch as the empire grew out of a league organized to retaliate against the Persians, any image of Athenian victory over the Persians might now also recall Athenian rule over her fellow Greeks.

The Acropolis' festivals reinforced these images of Athenian control. Paramount among these was the Greater Panathenaia, celebrated every five years over the course of about eight days. Panhellenic contests in poetry and athletics attracted people from around the Greek world, and metics took part freely in the festival's great procession along with manumitted slaves and barbarians.[13] But by later in the fifth century, Athens mandated participation in the event: in 425/4 BC Athens issued a decree requiring all cities of the empire to send a cow and suit of armor to the Greater Panathenaia (IG I³ 71), while decrees

addressed to specific cities, like Erythrai and Brea, included similar require-
ments (IG I³ 14; IG I³ 46).[14] The decree IG I³ 71 also stipulated reassessment of
the tribute every five years during the Greater Panathenaia.[15]

The festival's rituals, too, celebrated Athenian imperialism. The procession
paraded the cows and panoplies through the crowds who flocked to the city,
while a wheeled boat fitted out with Athena's peplos floated by as a symbol of
Athenian naval empire. The procession terminated on the Acropolis among
the very decrees mandating participation in the event.[16] Here, the cows required of the subject-allies were slaughtered in a massive sacrifice and the suits
of armor stored away in Athena's sanctuary.[17]

These associations were paramount when Asklepios sailed into Athens. The
decree requiring a cow and panoply for the Greater Panathenaia (IG I³ 71) had
been issued just five years earlier, and the first Greater Panathenaia at which it
was effective must have been that of 422/1 BC. Another decree, requiring the
appointment of tribute collectors (IG I³ 68), had been published on the Acropolis in 426. In addition, construction of the Temple of Athena Nike was underway in 420 or had only recently concluded.[18] The temple's friezes depicting
Greeks fighting Persians and even Greeks fighting fellow Greeks—the first
iconography that a visitor to the Acropolis encountered while ascending the
summit—set the scene for the larger theme of Athenian victory across the
Acropolis.[19] And construction may by 420 have begun on the Erechtheion,
named after Erechtheus, the legendary king of Athens who successfully de-
fended his city against a barbarian invasion that was later cast in terms of the
Persian assault.[20]

Asklepios' presence on the south slope of the Acropolis and the timing of
his arrival there in 420 BC, when imperialism was so much at issue that it had
led to civil war, made associations between Asklepios and empire inevitable.
These associations found reinforcement in the integration of his cult into the
cults of Dionysos Eleuthereus and Eleusinian Demeter.

Dionysos and Demeter

Before the arrival of Asklepios, Attic rituals linked Dionysos and Demeter.
Dionysos, albeit not as Eleuthereus, had a marked presence at Eleusis.[21] The
chorus of Sophocles' Antigone addresses Dionysos as "You who rule in the
all-welcoming folds of Eleusinian Demeter" (Ant. 1119–1121).[22] A red-figure
skyphos by Makron, dating to ca. 480 BC, depicts a personification of Eleusis,

along with Demeter, Persephone, Triptolemos, Eumolpos, Zeus, and Dionysos. Kevin Clinton, noting the equal size of the figures, has interpreted this vase and several others from the fourth century as indicating worship of Dionysos at Eleusis.[23]

Although no sanctuary to Dionysos has been identified at Eleusis, inscriptions from the fourth century mention celebrations of the Rural Dionysia there. One of these inscriptions attests to the importance of the Eleusinian Dionysia to the Athenian state: a chorus trainer who donated choruses at the Eleusinian Dionysia is praised for his *philotimia* towards both Eleusis and the Athenian demos (IG II² 1186).[24]

Dionysos also played a role in the Greater Mysteries. On the fifth day of the festival, an image of the god Iakchos escorted the initiates to Eleusis amid shouts of "*iakche*"; and when the initiates reached Eleusis, they celebrated Iakchos' arrival there (ὑποδοχή τοῦ ἰάκχου).[25] The names Iakchos and Dionysos (also known as Βάκχυς) were used interchangeably in literature as early as the mid-fifth century BC; in Sophocles' *Antigone*, the chorus calls Dionysos "Iakchos" (*Ant.* 1151).[26] Those who participated in the Mysteries must have sensed the similarity of Dionysos and Iakchos even if neither Dionysos himself nor his priests took part directly in the festival.[27]

Dionysos' presence at the Mysteries can be explained in part by the fact that he, like Demeter, was a god of mystery cult promising a better afterlife.[28] Moreover, both gave civilizing gifts to humans: Dionysos gave the vine and Demeter gave grain.[29] The timing of the Greater Mysteries and the City Dionysia within the Attic calendar enriched the agricultural connection between the two gods: the Greater Mysteries took place in Boedromion (late September–early October), six months after the City Dionysia. The gods of grain (which was sown soon after the Greater Mysteries) and the vine (which would have been budding in March at about the time of the City Dionysia) thus framed the Attic calendar.

Demeter's role in the cult of Dionysos Eleuthereus at Athens remains unattested, however, and Dionysos' presence at Eleusis is striking in contrast to a nearly complete absence of association between him and Demeter elsewhere in the Greek world.[30] The alignment of Dionysos and Demeter at Eleusis thus seems to have had more to do with local factors than general affinities between their cults. Accordingly, Asklepios' integration into both the Eleusinian Mysteries and the City Dionysia would have strengthened this particularly Athenian link between the cults of Dionysos and Demeter.

Dionysos Eleuthereus and the City Dionysia

The tract of land occupied by the sanctuary of Asklepios in Athens lay between the sanctuary of Dionysos to the east and a series of small sanctuaries of the Nymphs, Themis, and Aphrodite to the west.[31] Although the fifth-century extent of the sanctuaries of Asklepios and Dionysos is uncertain, by the fourth century, the growing monumentalization of both brought them into direct contact and alignment. The upper seats of the cavea of the Theater of Dionysos lay on level with the terraces of the Asklepieion, and the paving of the eastern terrace of the Asklepieion accommodated the cavea's curve.[32] Spatial proximity facilitated more than architectural contact between the two cults. A visitor to the fifth-century Acropolis would have encountered these sanctuaries in succession, as did Pausanias in the second century AD. In the larger "text" of the Acropolis, they were successive paragraphs, making associations readily available to the viewer.

Rituals reinforced these spatial links. The Asklepieia, one of Asklepios' two annual festivals in Athens, coincided with the City Dionysia. The events of the Asklepieia are poorly documented; we know only of a large sacrifice and παννυχίς, or all-night revelry. This festival was established probably soon after the arrival of Asklepios in 420.[33] According to Aeschines, the Asklepieia took place on the same day as the *proagon* to the City Dionysia, on Elaphebolion 8 (Aeschin. 3.66–67). During the *proagon*, poets, actors, and choruses of tragedies competing in the Dionysia stood in the Odeion of the sanctuary of Dionysos to announce the subjects of their plays.[34]

Why the state associated the cults of Asklepios and Dionysos Eleuthereus both spatially and ritually is a question almost never addressed in scholarship, and when it is mentioned, an underlying tone of surprise accompanies it. H. W. Parke, for example, writes, "In a curious way [the festival of Asklepios] *managed to intrude itself* into the Dionysia" (emphasis added).[35] The presence of Asklepios and his sons in plays like Sophocles' *Philoktetes* that were produced in the Theater of Dionysos augmented ties between the two cults, and some scholars have turned to drama to explain the connection.[36]

Early studies of Greek theater, for example, have argued that by late in the fifth century the cult of Asklepios at Epidauros had exerted strong influence on Athenian tragedy. As David Wiles explains, this model maintains that drama changed from something "agonistic or dialectical" to a "holistic, cathartic ideal embodied by Epidauros," which was in turn reflected in a shift from the rectangular theaters typical of Attic demes towards a circular theater "acousti-cally perfect for the paean, Apollo's lyre, and Homeric recitation."[37]

As Wiles and others have remarked, however, anachronism weakens these arguments. The theater building at Epidauros, said to exemplify the Apolline ideal, is a construction of the late fourth century.[38] To extrapolate the character of fifth-century Epidaurian poetry from the space it later occupied is problem-atic. Still more problematic is the suggestion that the fourth-century theater at Epidauros influenced the fifth-century Theater of Dionysos and Athenian trag-edy, much less the relationship between Asklepios and Dionysos there. Even the concept of tragic catharsis famously described by Aristotle (Poet. 1449b–1450a), which might be perceived as a healing process and thus akin to the cures of Asklepios, is unattested in the fifth century.

Athenian tragedy itself does address illness, often of the body politic. In Sophocles' Oedipus Tyrannus, a sickness attacks plant, animal, and human pro-creation at Thebes (the latter similar to the aition for the cult of Dionysos Eleuthereus described below; OT 1–77, esp. 59–69). Likewise in Aeschylus' Agamemnon, the eponymous hero announces upon his return to Argos that any disease befalling the city shall be treated with drugs, a scalpel, or cautery (Ag. 848–850). As the Agamemnon makes clear, not only is a healer necessary to treat the ailing body politic, but that healer ought to behave like a doctor.[39] Trage-dy's call for a physician to heal the ailing body politic may help to explain the link between tragedy and the doctor-god Asklepios, but there is no evidence that Asklepios had patients other than individuals until the late fourth cen-tury. Only then does the state thank him for the health and safety of the Athe-nian polis. As Jon Mikalson points out, moreover, this change marks a larger trend of thanking not just Asklepios but a number of the gods for the health and safety of Athens.[40]

To a limited extent, Dionysos himself functioned as healer. He was broadly associated with fertility; the grapevine, representative of plant growth, and the phallus were two of his most common symbols (although the primary function of the latter was apotropaic).[41] Dionysos could also inflict and cure illness. In one tradition, Dionysos Eleuthereus grew angry when the Athe-nians failed to receive him as a god, and so he afflicted the men of Athens with a genital disease until they fashioned phalluses to propitiate him (Schol. ad Ar. Ach. 243)—an aition for the procession of phalluses in the City Diony-sia. According to the fourth-century physician Mnesitheus, moreover, the Py-thian priestess ordered the Athenians to honor Dionysos as "Doctor" (Iatros), and by the fourth century Dionysos was also called Health-giver (Ὑγιάτης) and Healer (Παιώνιος).[42] Dionysos alleviated emotional suffering as well: in Euripides' *Bacchae* of 406 BC, he not only has the ability to reverse the madness he himself has instilled in Thebes, but his wine is said to be a *pharmakon* capable of easing grief and providing sleep and forgetfulness of daily cares (*Ba.* 278–283).

Given that Dionysos' healing role seems not to have been prominent in the fifth century, however, it is doubtful to have been the primary factor behind the alignment of Dionysos and Asklepios in Athens. Moreover, an explanation for this alignment based on healing raises the question why Dionysos, as opposed to a more overt healer, was linked to Asklepios. Given that all the gods had the power to heal, Asklepios could have been linked with any number of them. And, as we have seen, sanctuaries of Asklepios were often grafted onto sanctuaries of his father Apollo, a much more famous healer than Dionysos. Oddly, this is not the case in Athens where Apollo appears to have had no presence in the Asklepieion. Moreover, sanctuaries of Asklepios and Dionysos seem not to have been paired outside of Athens, which in itself, as in the case of Dionysos and Demeter, suggests a local reason for their Athenian alignment.[43]

The Sanctuary of Dionysos Eleuthereus

Anyone standing in the sanctuary of Dionysos Eleuthereus had only to gaze up to the summit of the Acropolis to see the temple of Athena Parthenos, goddess of the Panathenaia and of the empire, dominating the view. This was not true for sanctuaries on the north and west slopes of the Acropolis, where other structures and the elevation of the summit obstructed one's view of the Parthenon.[44]

By 420 BC, the sanctuary of Dionysos included the Theater of Dionysos, a small temple, and the Odeion. The Theater of Dionysos was not yet the monumental stone structure it would become in the fourth century (as Rush Rehm so aptly describes, its fifth-century incarnation "was less a building than what we would call landscape architecture"), but its wooden bleachers utilized a natural concavity in the hillside to provide seating for at least all of the male citizen population as well as notable visitors.[45] The focal point of this cavea was the orchestra, behind which stood a modest temple of Dionysos dating to the Archaic period. But the most striking monumental element of the sanctuary in the late fifth century was the Odeion, whose architecture, as noted above, resembled that of the Telesterion at Eleusis.

A large, roofed, almost square hall to the east of the orchestra, the Odeion housed musical contests, dramatic events, and even court proceedings.[46] Its building history is debated by ancient sources. Vitruvius attributes it to Themistocles; Plutarch to Pericles (Vitr. 5.9.1; Plu. *Per.* 13.6). Both versions agree, however, that the structure celebrated Greece's victory over Persia. Vitruvius says that the posts supporting the roof were taken from Persian warships, and Plutarch and Pausanias remark that the structure was built to resemble the Persian king's tent (Vitr. 5.9.1; Plu. *Per.* 13.5–6; Paus. 1.20.4).[47]

As a Persian victory monument, and like victory monuments on the summit of the Acropolis, the Odeion by the later fifth century could carry connotations also of Athenian dominance and thereby share in the reflexive text of empire published across the Acropolis. If Plutarch is right, the very financing of the project invited such connotations: he states that tribute from Athens' allies helped fund its construction (Plut. *Per.* 12.1–5). Plutarch also reports that under Pericles' direction, musical contests belonging to the Greater Panathenaia were staged in the Odeion (Plut. *Per.* 13.11). The Panathenaia, itself so heavily imbued with imperial overtones, drew the sanctuary of Dionysos more fully into the text of imperial references.[48]

The City Dionysia

The strongest link between the sanctuary of Dionysos and Athenian empire resided not in its architecture, however, but in the rituals of the City Dionysia. Taking place annually over a period of five days, this festival in honor of Dionysos Eleuthereus drew attention to Athens' position as head of a vast empire.[49]

John Winkler has proposed that numerous elements of the festival's dramatic competitions reflected and celebrated the polis, including such practicalities as the seating of the audience by demes and the military training of the chorus. Simon Goldhill elucidates how rituals that preceded the dramatic competitions also celebrated Athens.[50] Citizens who had made significant contributions to the city were awarded gold crowns, and children of men killed in war were brought onto the stage; these latter, it was announced, had been raised and trained by the city to fight on its behalf. And Athens' generals poured libations prior to performances in the Theater of Dionysos. All of these rituals eulogized the power—past, present, and future—of the city in much the same way as did the public funeral held each year to commemorate Athenians who had died in war.[51] These rituals functioned also as displays of Athenian military strength and thus acquired new meaning in the years around 420 BC as Athens attempted to stifle insurrection within its empire.

Other aspects of the festival more explicitly articulated Athenian empire. According to the slander-wary Dikaiopolis in Aristophanes' *Acharnians* of 425 BC, an Athenian must be very careful what he says during the City Dionysia since more foreigners than usual are present in Athens (*Ach.* 496–509).[52] One reason for this influx from out of town was the schedule of tribute payment: Athens decreed that cities of the empire pay imperial tribute by the start of the City Dionysia.[53] The Athenian state thus coordinated the financing of empire with this Athenian festival, much as it coordinated the reassessment of tribute with the Greater Panathenaia.

Imperial tribute was integrated into the very rituals of the City Dionysia. Paraded into the Theater of Dionysos and laid out, talent by talent, across the orchestra (Isoc. 8.82), it became yet another staged spectacle that brought home, quite literally, the message of Athenian imperialism to residents and visitors alike.[54] Moreover, Athens required at least one imperial colony to send a carved wooden phallus for the procession of the City Dionysia, in addition to a cow and suit of armor for the Greater Panathenaia (Brea: IG I³ 46). Unlike most processions, which moved from the center of the city to its periphery, the processions of the Greater Panathenaia and City Dionysia moved from the periphery towards the center, terminating on the Acropolis (Panathenaia) or its slopes (Dionysia) amidst numerous indications of empire.[55] Reciprocal in form and function, these processions, whose movement resembled the journey of representatives of the allied states from the periphery of the empire to its ruling head, marked the centrality and power of Athens.[56]

This climate, steeped in symbols and rituals recalling Athenian empire, proved conducive also to negotiating imperial business. Around 430 BC, Athens issued a decree attempting to restrict Macedonian interference in Methone with the stipulation that, should Macedonia not cooperate, both Macedonia and Methone would be required to send envoys to the City Dionysia to negotiate (IG I³ 61). This decree stood in the Theater of Dionysos and featured Athena, goddess of the empire, on its relief.[57] In addition, Athens and Sparta ratified the preliminary measures of the Peace of Nicias during the City Dionysia of 421 BC and agreed to renew the treaty each year at this festival.[58] Thus in 420, the cult of Dionysus Eleuthereus overtly celebrated Athenian empire. The same is true for the cult of Eleusinian Demeter.

Eleusinian Demeter and the Mysteries

Each year the Epidauria celebrated Asklepios' arrival in Athens during the Eleusinian Mysteries. The civic calendar thereby fixed Asklepios' association with the cult of Eleusinian Demeter and ensured that the association would be reinforced on an annual basis.

The alignment of Asklepios and Demeter, unlike that of Asklepios and Dionysos, appeared in ritual, art, and topography in many places in the Greek world. Christa Benedum has mapped these alignments at Epidauros, Sikyon, Troezen, Hermione, Paros, and Aegina, to list but a few.[59] She accounts for the coordination of these two gods in terms of their salvific powers. While Asklepios heals the living, Demeter aids with the afterlife. Thus, both mediate the life-death border and provide mitigated triumph over death. Both, moreover, focus on the individual: Demeter brings a different afterlife to those who undergo initiation into her Mysteries, just as Asklepios brings health to those who sleep in his sanctuaries.[60]

Benedum's explanation for the cultic alignment of Asklepios and Demeter is compelling, especially since it accounts for the prevalence of the phenomenon. But, as Robert Parker notes, none of the evidence cited by Benedum for the alignment of Asklepios and Demeter predates the arrival of Asklepios in Athens.[61] Thus, while health in a general sense, especially as an extension of salvific benefits, may help explain many of these instances, it cannot be used as paradigmatic of the association in Athens.

Other general characteristics link the two gods. Both, for example, offer civilizing gifts to mankind: Demeter offers agriculture and Asklepios medicine. Aelius Aristides would even compare Machaon and Podaleirios (Asklepios' sons) to Triptolemos (Demeter's son) as propagators of medicine and agriculture, respectively (*Or.* 38.15). The pseudo-Hippocratic letters would do the same for Hippocrates (*Ep.* 9). These traditions, however, appear relatively late in the historical record.[62]

Athens may have been responding to any or all of these affinities when it aligned the cults of Demeter and Asklepios in 420 BC, but the so-called First-Fruits decree (IG I³ 78) suggests that another aspect of the cult of Eleusinian Demeter prominent at the time influenced the alignment. This decree, issued by Athens probably in the 420s BC, details provisions for the offering of ἀπαρχαί, or first fruits, to Demeter and Kore.[63] Individuals traditionally offered first fruits, or a portion of the annual harvest, to local deities. These first fruits could be combined to represent the offering of an entire community. The imperial tribute to Athena, for example, was a first fruits offering collected city by city, as attested by the tribute quota lists. Demeter's role as goddess of grain made her an obvious and doubtless longstanding recipient of first fruits of the grain harvest in many Greek cities.

Another decree (IG I³ 6), dating to ca. 460 BC, provides the earliest evidence of first fruits offered to Demeter at Eleusis.[64] According to this decree, issued by Eleusis, the proceeds from the first fruits (that is, the money made from sale of the grain) were to be stored in Athena's sanctuary on the Athenian Acropolis and to be used at the discretion of the Athenians. Athens thus reaped the benefits of Eleusinian finances.

As opposed to IG I³ 6, the First-Fruits decree demands that the entire empire offer first fruits to Eleusinian Demeter (IG I³ 78, lines 14–24). Such a mandate is closely akin to Athens' requirement that the empire pay annual tribute to Athena, that this tribute be brought to Athens every year at the time of the City Dionysia, and that all cities of the empire send a cow and suit of armor to the Greater Panathenaia. Like these other mandates, the First-Fruits decree is an expression of Athenian control over its empire. Significantly, the particular clause governing members of the empire mentions neither "tradition" nor the "oracular response of Delphi," invoked four times elsewhere in the decree to buttress Athens' authority in making these provisions. The absence of both here suggests that Athens could not claim sanction by either tradition or the Delphic oracle for requiring first fruits from its allies.

Beyond her own empire, Athens urged all the Greeks to contribute first fruits to Eleusinian Demeter (IG I³ 78, lines 24–34); and for this measure the decree did assert sanction by both tradition and Delphi. Only an Athens confident in its position would exert its influence over the entire Greek world. About this decree Robert Parker writes, "It may well have been traditional for a tithe of crops to be sent to Eleusis by the Attic demes . . . ; but it was doubtless only at the height of her political and cultic hegemony that Athens, with the support of the Delphic oracle, could press her claims on the rest of the Greek world."[65]

Athens thus exploited the prestige of the cult of Eleusinian Demeter to promote Athenian empire. It should not be surprising that the rider to the First-Fruits decree contains a scheme for another first fruits offering, this one of olive oil, presumably in honor of Athena, who gave the olive to Athens (IG I³ 78, lines 59–61). Although the proposal evidently never passed, as Parker comments, "It is revealing that it was made."[66] It reveals Athenian ambition and confidence but also a particular interest in celebrating Athenian empire via Demeter and Athena. Since both had large panhellenic cults in Athens, they were obvious gods to promote the empire.

Other Athenian rituals further associated these two goddesses with one another and with empire. The Panathenaic procession, for example, passed by the Eleusinion and thereby wove Eleusinian Demeter into the web of imperial references that crowded the Acropolis.[67] Moreover, during the Greater Mysteries a herald visited Athena's priestess on the Acropolis to announce the arrival at the Eleusinion of the "holy things" from Eleusis.[68] Demeter was thus subordinated to the patron goddess of the empire. And, as mentioned above, proceeds from the sale of Eleusinian first fruits were housed in Athena's sanctuary on the Acropolis (attested in IG I³ 6 and again in IG I³ 386 of 408/7 BC), presumably alongside the imperial tribute. The integration of Asklepios into Demeter's cult in 420 BC cannot have been without studied implications for Asklepios.

It makes sense that the cults of Dionysos Eleuthereus and Eleusinian Demeter would accord in the celebration and maintenance of Athenian empire in 420, inasmuch as the festivals of both cults attracted huge panhellenic audiences and thus served as ideal venues for advertising widely Athens' accomplishments and aspirations. It is perhaps significant in this regard that at Athens the largest festivals of Dionysos and Demeter marked the beginning and end of the annual military campaigning season (late March–early October). Both festivals also celebrated Athens' territorial expansion, as many scholars have discussed. Much as the Mysteries marked Athens' acquisition of Eleusis on the border with Megara, the City Dionysia in honor of Dionysos Eleuthereus marked the acquisition of Eleutherai on the border with Boeotia.[69] By 420 even the Greater Panathenaia could be viewed as a celebration of territorial expansion, in this case of the borders not of Attica but of Athenian empire.

The alignment of Asklepios with the Acropolis and Greater Panathenaia, with the sanctuary of Dionysos Eleuthereus and the City Dionysia, and with the Eleusinion and Eleusinian Mysteries suggests an elaborate orchestration capable of evoking particular associations. Each of these links alone may not be significant, but the accumulation of evidence is striking. While factors such as health and the agricultural cycle help explain this orchestration, the ties to Athenian empire are impossible to ignore. Athenians must have viewed the importation of Asklepios as relevant to imperial policy, and particularly to the acquisition of new territory.

CHAPTER SIX

Asklepios and Athenian Empire

The history of fifth-century Athenian religion is inseparable
from the history of Athenian political and social aspirations, and
the centrality of religion . . . requires us to evaluate the two side
by side.

Robert Garland, Introducing New Gods, 171

Epidauros, located on the northern coast of the Akte peninsula, faces the
Saronic Gulf (Fig. 6.1). The strategic importance of this gulf and its numerous harbors had long been apparent to the Greeks. During the Persian Wars, for instance, the Greek fleet assembled at the harbor of Pogon in the
Troezenia before sailing to victory at Salamis in 480 BC.[1] The advantages of the
gulf and particularly its harbor at Epidauros would draw increasing attention
from Athens as its naval power expanded.

Epidauros and Athens in the Peloponnesian Wars

During the so-called First Peloponnesian War (460–451, and 446 BC), Athens
fought cities of the Saronic Gulf including Epidauros (Thucy. 1.105.1; Diod.Sic.
11.78). War began when Athens attacked Halieis, a city on the southern coast of
the Akte peninsula. Troops from Epidauros, Sikyon, and Corinth repelled the
attack. As Michael Jameson observes, the concerted and timely effort of the Peloponnesian cities suggests their awareness of Athenian interest in the area.[2]

By the start of the next Peloponnesian War, Athenian interest had expanded
much beyond the Saronic Gulf to include all of the Peloponnese. Athens' quick-
est route into the Peloponnese was from Piraeus, just southwest of Athens,
across the Saronic Gulf, to Epidauros. In 430, Athens ravaged the territories of
several cities on the Akte peninsula (Thucy. 2.56.4–5).[3] The territory of Epidauros was the first to be attacked, but Athens did not succeed in taking the

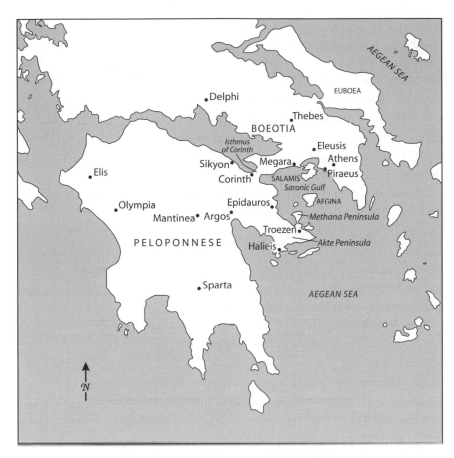

Figure 6.1. Map of Central Grace and the Peloponnese. (Map by Christopher Brest.)

city itself. In 425, Athens, having taken the smaller peninsula, Methana, built a wall to separate it from the rest of the Akte. Athens also established a garrison on Methana and used this garrison to raid the territories of Epidauros and other cities (Thucy. 4.45.2). These raids presumably recurred for a number of years, perhaps until the Peace of Nicias.[4]

In 421 BC, Athens and Sparta declared the so-called Peace of Nicias, but fighting would resume between the allies of Athens and Sparta in less than two years. It was in this two-year period that the cult of Asklepios was brought to Athens from Epidauros.

The importance of Epidauros to Athens becomes especially clear in events subsequent to the Peace of Nicias. When hostilities resumed, the first city attacked was Epidauros. During the summer of 419, the Athenian general Alcibiades convinced the Argives, who had just formed an alliance with Athens, to attack Epidauros, which was still allied with Sparta (Thucy. 5.53). According to Thucydides, the real motive for this act was to bring Epidauros under the control of Argos and Athens (Thucy. 5.53.1).[5] Capturing Epidauros would, in part, facilitate communication between Athens and Argos: rather than having to sail all the way around Cape Skyllaion, the easternmost point of the Akte peninsula, Athenians could sail from Aegina to Epidauros and then travel over land directly west to Argos. Argos thus attacked Epidauros, precipitating a war between them. Athens supported Argos in the war.[6]

The following winter (419/18 BC), Sparta sent troops north by sea to support the Epidaurians in their war against Argos. Argos complained that Athens had allowed Spartan troops into Epidauros past Athenian garrisons (Thucy. 5.56.1–2). According to the terms of the Peace of Nicias, enemy troops were not allowed to pass through allied territory without consent of all the allies (Thucy. 5.47.5). With this act, the peace was compromised and the Argive war on Epidauros continued with Athenian support.[7]

Later in 418 BC, Sparta won a major victory at Mantineia. Fear of Spartan power shifted the allegiance of some Argives, who not only negotiated a peace with Epidauros but persuaded Athens to do the same (Thucy. 5.80). The cities of the Akte peninsula were further encouraged by Athenian defeat in Sicily in 413 BC and remained active supporters of Sparta throughout the Peloponnesian War and well into the fourth century BC. As a result, Athens made no successful advances in the area for many years.

Not until the mid-fourth century BC did Athenian military activity in the Akte peninsula resume.[8] In 365, Spartan dominance in the peninsula ended when Thebes attacked the northern Peloponnese. That year Epidauros made peace with Thebes (Isoc. 6.91; Xen. Hell. 7.4.9). Meanwhile, Athens also negotiated a peace with Epidauros in the hope of establishing a bloc against Theban dominance (Arist. Rhet. 1411a.11). That Athens made a treaty with Epidauros as soon as Epidauros was out of Spartan control indicates how important this city continued to be.

Athenian interest in Epidauros, particularly during the Peloponnesian War, was due to several geographical factors. First, the harbor at Epidauros afforded safe and convenient anchorage for the Athenian navy; moreover, it was the port of entry into the Peloponnese closest to Athens. For a naval power like Athens, Epidauros was especially appealing. Second, Epidauros was the city on the Akte peninsula nearest the Isthmus of Corinth—the only land route into and out of the Peloponnese. Control of Epidauros would thus enable Athens to safeguard its own troops' entry into the Peloponnese while also preventing Peloponnesian troops from invading Attica, an annual calamity for Athens during the war.[9]

Furthermore, Epidauros was a powerful city, and thanks to the cult of Asklepios, increasingly wealthy, as Alison Burford has documented.[10] According to Λ. W. Gomme, it was the second most important city on the Akte peninsula after Argos.[11] The impact of its participation in acts of defiance against Athens (such as the Corcyrean affair and Megarian revolt, which precipitated the war) must have been great.[12] Moreover, its defeat of Epidauros would have weakened Peloponnesian confidence drastically during the war. A nearby city like Corinth, for example, would surely have felt exposed if Epidauros allied with Athens, and especially if Argos joined the alliance.

Thucydides writes that the real cause of the Peloponnesian War was fear of the growing dominance of Athens (Thucy. 1.23.5–6).[13] In other words, it was a war about Athenian empire. The ability of Athens to maintain its empire depended in large part on gaining control of the Peloponnese; forging closer ties with Epidauros was key to achieving this goal, and the importation of the Epidaurian cult of Asklepios presented one way to forge such ties.

The Peace of Nicias and Epidaurian Asklepios

When Asklepios arrived in Athens in 420 BC, Athens and Sparta had been at war for ten years and at peace for one. By the terms of the Peace of Nicias, Athens and Sparta were to remain at peace for fifty years (Thucy. 5.23), but Thucydides, who saw Athens and Sparta as engaged in one long war lasting from 431 to 404 BC, describes the peace as doomed to fail (Thucy. 5.26.1–2).[14]

Several factors made it difficult to maintain the peace. According to Thucydides, those factors had less to do with Athenian and Spartan interest in resuming the war than with displeasure among Sparta's allies over the terms of the peace (Thucy. 5.29.3). Corinth, Boeotia, Elis, and Megara had all voted against the peace in 421, not least because the final clause authorized Athens and Sparta together to amend the treaty without consulting their allies. Aggrieved, these cities took steps to form an independent league under the leadership of Argos.

Although this league did not materialize, the actions of Boeotia in particular proved fatal to the peace. In 420, Boeotia manipulated Sparta into concluding a separate alliance with them (Thucy. 5.39.2–3). When Athens learned of this alliance, negotiations between Athens and Sparta broke down. Athens threatened to ally with Argos, Mantineia, and Elis unless (1) Sparta severed its alliance with Boeotia and (2) the Boeotians agreed to the Peace of Nicias. Sparta refused (Thucy. 5.46.4); the new quadruple alliance including Athens, Elis, Mantineia, and Argos was formed (Thucy. 5.47),[15] and Athens and Sparta no longer exchanged embassies to negotiate. Although the Peace of Nicias was still nominally in effect, it was fast eroding.

However, frequent communication and negotiation between Sparta and Athens in 421 and 420 indicate that these two powers were for some time interested in maintaining peace. Thucydides records that in the summer of 421/20 alone there were numerous conferences between the two cities and "peace and exchange with each other" (ἡσυχία ἦν καὶ ἔφοδοι παρ' ἀλλήλους, Thucy. 5.35.7–8). The following winter, more discussions took place between Athens and Sparta while other powers, like Boeotia, continued to stir up suspicion and animosity (Thucy. 5.39.2). Even when the Boeotians manipulated Sparta into accepting an alliance with them, Sparta continued sending embassies to Athens in the spring of 420, apparently hoping to settle the matter amicably. Not even a ruse on the part of the Athenian general Alcibiades to compromise the integrity of Sparta's envoys derailed the peace. Instead, Athens sent envoys back to Sparta to continue to negotiate (Thucy. 5.43–46; Plut. Nik. 10). When finally even these discussions failed, Athens allied with Argos and all further negotiation ceased (Thucy. 5.47).

It is difficult to determine from Thucydides' narrative the exact timing of final negotiations between Athens and Sparta, but Asklepios probably came to Athens soon after these talks had ended. Importing any cult, much less a well-established panhellenic cult, was not an instantaneous matter and must have required some period of negotiation between Athens and Epidauros. These negotiations were probably carried out while Athens and Sparta were at peace, but whether they still expected to avoid war is uncertain. In either event, the importation of Asklepios promised Athens a strong position in relation to Epidauros, and thereby also the Peloponnese.

Athens, Cults, and Politics in the Fifth Century

Sources since antiquity have claimed that Athens, as well as many other Greek states, adopted and adapted cults for what we consider political ends. For example, the sixth-century tyrant Peisistratos is often said to have manipulated cults, festivals, and sanctuaries to garner popular support for himself and to promote allegiance to Athens. He is credited with building the first stone temple to Athena on the Acropolis, reorganizing the Panathenaia, founding or re-founding the City Dionysia, building a predecessor to the temple to Zeus Olympios, constructing sanctuaries in the Agora, rebuilding the initiation building (Telesterion) at Eleusis, purifying Delos and building a temple there, and tailoring the myths of Herakles and Theseus.[16] Peisistratos may not in fact have instigated many of these measures, but that Greeks of later centuries thought he did indicates that what we might label "religious" innovation was often ascribed to the interests of the state.

This ancient pattern has largely shaped modern perceptions of sixth- and fifth-century Athenian religion. Regarding the fifth century, the period after tyranny had been overthrown and democracy established, scholars focus on foreign policy as the most prevalent factor behind developments in cults and festivals. The Persian Wars in particular are considered a primary cause for introducing new cults or expanding preexisting ones.[17] These wars apparently sparked changes in the cults of Athena Nike, Theseus, Pan, Artemis Aristoboule, Boreas, Poseidon (at Sounion), Nemesis (at Rhamnous), Apollo (at Phaleron), among others, most often as a means of thanking the various deities for help in the war.[18] Other wars and other matters of foreign and domestic policy are likewise said to have driven developments in fifth-century Athenian cult.

The importation of Asklepios, by stark contrast, is never cast in the light of state interests. In order to better appreciate the exclusion of Asklepios from this interpretive model, it will be helpful to look briefly at two deities, Theseus and Bendis, and how their myths and cults are said to have been manipulated in response to Athenian foreign policy.

Athenians credited their legendary king Theseus with bringing much of Attica under Athenian control.[19] As a young man, Theseus journeyed from Troezen to Athens and killed five menacing opponents along the way.[20] These five acts, known as his labors, had developed into a consistent system by 510 BC; potters were painting the series of labors onto their wares and sculptors soon began carving them onto metopes.[21]

The five labors all took place on the Isthmus of Corinth or near Eleusis (the first near the location of the Isthmian games, the second and third near Megara, and the fourth and fifth near Eleusis). All these were places where, at least according to ancient tradition, Athens had vied for territorial control and won it under Theseus. In the late sixth century and early fifth century, Athens was trying to (re)gain control of some of these same territories, especially the Megarid.[22] Evident in the labors of Theseus, therefore, was a tradition of Attic synoecism and hope for further expansion. The myth of Theseus affirmed what Athens already controlled, namely Eleusis, and provided mythic validation for its claims to further territory.

The Theseus cycle later expanded to include a sixth encounter at Epidauros against an opponent named Periphetes, but exactly when the tradition of this labor developed is uncertain.[23] It is tempting to associate this encounter with the importance of Epidauros to Athens during the Peloponnesian Wars. Just as the importation of Asklepios reflected Athenian foreign policy regarding Epidauros, the Theseus cycle may have been tailored to do the same.

The formulation of Theseus' labors into a consistent pattern at the turn of the fifth century, when Athens was not only promoting the role of Theseus in its shift from tyranny to democracy but was contending over some of the very locations these labors entailed, cannot be coincidental. As Henry Walker comments, the Theseus cycle is "a visual representation of the perennial Athenian dream of ruling the Isthmus. . . . It is a dream that lasts from Solon to the Peloponnesian War."[24]

The introduction of Bendis into Piraeus around 430 BC likewise reflects Athenian interests at the time.[25] According to Thucydides, Thrace was a focus of Athenian interest for many years prior to her arrival (Thucy. 2.29.4). Its allure lay largely in its geography and wealth. Rich in natural resources, particularly timber, necessary for maintaining the large Athenian fleet, Thrace sits near the Hellespont, through which all trade north to the Black Sea had to pass. Furthermore, Athens had allies and colonies on the Thracian coast (e.g., Amphipolis and Brea).

Thucydides records several instances of Athenian intervention in the area. In 432, the Athenians besieged Potideia after it revolted, and they fought against Perdiccas, king of Macedonia. In 431, Athens concluded a treaty with both Perdiccas and Sitalkes of Thrace (Thucy. 2.29.5–6), and for several years Sitalkes aided Athens. During this period of peace and amicability, Bendis arrived in Piraeus. Regarding the treaty of 431 between Athens and Sitalkes, Martin Nilsson writes, "The reception of the Thracian goddess into the Athenian state cult has its appropriate place precisely in connection with this highly political event." In this reading, Athens' importation of Bendis was a way to consolidate its alliance with Thrace.[26]

So apparently obvious is the Athenian state's manipulation of cults and deities to articulate and advance its political interests that Nilsson states, "The transference of cults is *a well-known expedient* to unite an incorporated district with the ruling city" (emphasis added), and Robert Garland sums up developments in fifth-century Athenian cults thus: "The conclusion *seems irresistible* that the Demos utilized religious worship for the furthering of its foreign policy. . . . In domestic as well as in foreign policy, a state's gods were deeply implicated in the advancement of its aims" (emphasis added).[27]

Are scholars pressing the political motives too far? It is possible; we should not reduce the significance of cults and festivals merely to issues of military and foreign policy. But in the case of Asklepios, military and foreign interests remain entirely unexplored.

Negotiating Empire

After years of warfare, the Peace of Nicias afforded an opportunity for increased diplomatic maneuvering, and Athens reacted by importing Epidauros' signature god as a way of forging an alliance with a city critical to Athenian success against Peloponnesian aggression.

Several signs imply that Asklepios' importation was a cooperative endeavor between Athens and Epidauros, as Kevin Clinton has observed. First, a sacred law of the late fifth century from the Athenian Agora attests to the involvement of Epidaurian officials in the festival celebrating Asklepios' arrival, a tradition that probably reflects their involvement in the importation itself in 420 (Agora inv. no. I 7471). The presence of these Epidaurian officials indicates that Epidauros approved of bringing Asklepios to Athens. Athens did not abduct Asklepios; rather, Athens negotiated his importation.[28]

More striking as evidence for cooperation is the name of the festival commemorating Asklepios' arrival: the Epidauria. While cults often took their names from locales, few took them from foreign locales. There was thus no tradition compelling Athenians to name this festival "Epidauria"; they could as easily have called it the "Asklepieia," for instance, along the lines of the Dionysia.[29] Instead, Athens chose to publicize the Epidaurian origin of the cult and to memorialize it each year in the name of this annual cult festival.

Why Athens chose to do so is uncertain. Perhaps Athens hoped that the name would lend prestige to its own cult, given the popularity of the Epidaurian sanctuary. But the name may also have served as a declaration of Athens' aspirations for alliance with Epidauros. It is not difficult to imagine the benefits Athens could reap from such alliance: use of a strategic harbor, easier access to the Peloponnese, and all that such access entailed for control of the Peloponnese.

But what would Epidauros have hoped to gain from the bargain? Having Athens as an ally may have been viewed as a self-defensive measure. Athens was the perpetrator of many attacks on Epidauros in the 420s, and an amicable relationship with Athens lessened the risk that Epidauros would be the target of future aggression. Alliance with Athens likewise promised Epidauros a greater sense of security on all fronts, especially against powerful, inimical neighbors like Argos.

Economic reasons must also have factored into the Epidaurian decision. Athens promoted Epidauros in at least two ways: naming the festival "Epidauria" called attention to Epidauros, while integration of the Epidaurian god into two major panhellenic festivals likewise boosted his hometown's exposure.[30] Any advertising (intentional or not) that Athens did for the Epidaurian cult increased the volume of visitors to Epidauros, and consequently also the cult's finances. More visitors meant more offerings. Had Athens hoped to detract panhellenic business from Epidauros, its plan clearly backfired. Most visitors to the Athenian Asklepieion were Athenians; the cult at Epidauros, on the other hand, continued to flourish and draw individuals from around the Greek world, and engaged in a vast building program in the fourth century. Furthermore, Robert Garland proposes that sanctuaries founded from Epidauros contributed a percentage of their fees to the mother sanctuary. If so, Athens could have been making financial contributions to Epidauros as early as the fifth century.[31]

It is thus possible to see why Epidauros would have found friendly ties with Athens advantageous, especially vis-à-vis the cult of Asklepios, and vice versa. But if Athens was indeed interested in alliance with Epidauros, why did Athens take part in Argive aggression against Epidauros in 419 BC, within a year of importing Asklepios?

The decision to pursue a peaceful alliance with an enemy state can hardly have been a unilateral one for either Athens or Epidauros in the charged, wartime politics of the late 420s, and the attack on Epidauros in 419 points to factionalism on the Athenian side. About the attack Thucydides writes, "It seemed best to Alcibiades and the Argives, if possible, to acquire Epidauros" (Thucy. 5.53).[32] The role of Alcibiades in this effort is suspicious. He was among those Athenians opposed to peace with Sparta (Thucy. 5.43). Thucydides attributes Alcibiades' anti-Spartan stance partly to his wounded pride. Alcibiades had hoped to become proxenos to Sparta, an office that his grandfather had held and later given up (Thucy. 5.89; cf. Plut. Alc. 14). When Sparta prepared to negotiate peace with Athens in 421, however, it chose to do so not through Alcibiades, as

Alcibiades had expected, but through the Athenian generals Nicias and Laches (Thucy. 5.43).

Thus slighted, Alcibiades set about convincing his fellow Athenians that the peace was a bad idea because Sparta was untrustworthy. In the spring of 420, a year after the peace had been negotiated (and still prior to the importation of Asklepios, who would arrive the following autumn), Alcibiades argued that Sparta would attack Argos and thereby leave Athens isolated unless Athens allied itself with Argos (Thucy. 5.43). He must have known that his rhetoric would appeal to ongoing Athenian concerns over the northeastern Peloponnese. When Spartan envoys arrived in Athens that same spring to dissuade Athens from allying with Argos, Alcibiades sabotaged their efforts by tricking them into appearing unwilling and unprepared to participate fully in negotiations (Thucy. 5.45; Plut. Nic. 10). At the same time, Alcibiades was secretly urging Argos to ally with Athens.

Alcibiades' actions as a newly elected general in 419 demonstrate even more clearly his intention to stir up hostilities against Sparta and provoke Sparta into breaking the peace. In the spring of 419, Alcibiades led an ostentatious expedition across the northern Peloponnese with a largely Peloponnesian army, to flaunt Athens' presence there at a moment of Spartan weakness (Thucy. 5.52.2).[33] That summer, Alcibiades engineered the Argive attack on Epidauros; Sparta responded in 418 by sending a garrison to help its ally. When Argos complained that Spartan troops had traveled through Athenian territory without the latter's permission, Alcibiades convinced the Athenians to amend the inscription bearing the peace. It now read that the Spartans did not keep their oaths (Thucy. 5.56).

For Alcibiades, who understood the importance of Epidauros to Athens' position, the alliance forged between the gods of Athens and Epidauros was simply inadequate. Epidauros had to be brought fully over to Athens' side even if that meant renewed military aggression against Epidauros. Athens could not attack Epidauros without breaking the peace, but Argos could, since it had not been a party to the peace.

There were thus at least two factions within Athens debating how best to bring Epidauros into alliance. Alcibiades' anti-Spartan faction favored the use of force against Epidauros in order to give Athens a more secure link with Argos and more control generally over their alliance partner. Another faction, interested in preserving peace with Sparta, pursued alliance with Epidauros through the importation of Asklepios. The latter faction got its way long enough to import the cult, but the anti-Spartan one prevailed by convincing

Argos to attack Epidauros. The war between Argos and Epidauros that followed this attack in 419 quickly eroded any amicable relations between Epidauros and Athens.

So far in this discussion, those favoring peaceful alliance with Epidauros have remained anonymous; but Nicias and Laches, the architects of the peace, probably numbered among them. Another name that almost certainly belongs to the faction is Kallias (III). This Kallias was a leader of the Kerykes and proxenos for Sparta at about the time of Asklepios' importation.[34] Clinton has proposed that Kallias participated in the negotiations to bring Asklepios to Athens. As proxenos for Sparta, he would have been on favorable terms with Epidauros and thus in a good position to negotiate between Epidauros and Athens.[35] His role in the importation would also accord with his prominent position in the Kerykes, the priestly family of Eleusinian Demeter that welcomed Asklepios to Athens.

Disagreement between Kallias and Alcibiades on how best to handle Epidauros also fits a larger pattern of hostility between the two. Alcibiades had married Kallias' sister Hipparete sometime before 424, but it is said that he so badly mistreated her that she tried to divorce him (Pseudo-Andocides, *Against Alcibiades* 13; Plut. *Alc.* 8). Alcibiades is also said to have planned Kallias' murder in order to acquire his wealth. Other antagonisms erupted later: given that Kallias was a member of the Kerykes, he may have been involved in the accusations brought against Alcibiades in 415 for parodying the Eleusinian Mysteries; and, according to Thucydides, the Kerykes opposed Alcibiades' recall in 408 (Thucy. 8.53.2). Whether these animosities had anything to do with these two men's opposing views on Epidauros remains speculative.

Despite their opposing views on Epidauros, Alcibiades would not necessarily have opposed the importation of Asklepios. He and many other Athenians may have hoped that if Asklepios were given a warm enough welcome, his allegiances would at least be divided between Epidauros and Athens, if not squarely on the side of the latter. And if Asklepios were happy in his new home, he might even allow the Athenians to conquer his first one. Such a strategy, so the story goes, had worked for Solon: according to Plutarch, because Solon propitiated Salamis' heroes, Athens succeeded in taking the island (Plut. *Sol.* 9).[36] Bringing Asklepios to Athens thus had its advantages for both factions.

Asklepios and the Kerykes in 418 BC

Although Alcibiades' anti-Spartan faction ultimately prevailed and relations between Epidauros and Athens deteriorated, the efforts of the pro-peace faction left an indelible mark on the ritual landscape of Athens. Epidaurian Asklepios kept his prestigious position on the Acropolis, his prime-time festivals, and his devoted worshippers. Not even open hostility between Epidauros and Athens in 418 could threaten his position—or could it?

In Chapter 4, I argued that the land dispute of 418 mentioned on the Telemachos monument reflects actions taken by the Kerykes against another, unnamed party meddling in the affairs of Asklepios' sanctuary. While I favor this interpretation, another possibility emerges from events in 418. As we have seen, war broke out between Argos and Epidauros in 419. In the summer of 418, just before the Battle of Mantinea, Epidauros took advantage of the Argives' divided attentions to invade Argos (Thucy. 5.75). In response, Athenian forces that had come to fight at Mantinea marched against Epidauros, walled the city, and left a garrison behind. Only when Argos finally decided to sign a treaty with Sparta the following winter did Athens withdraw the garrison (Thucy. 5.80).

Perhaps Epidauros' attack on Argos, an Athenian ally, soured the Kerykes' enthusiasm for Asklepios. As a result, the statement on the Telemachos monument that "the Kerykes disputed the land" may indicate that the Kerykes tried to oust the Epidaurian god from his Athenian home out of anger or embarrassment over their longstanding support of him.

But, even had the Kerykes wanted to remove Asklepios, there was little chance that by 418, two years into his residence, they alone could have succeeded in evicting him. Asklepios had become so entrenched in Athens, and the demand for his healing was so great, that no matter how Epidauros behaved, Asklepios was now a favorite citizen of Athens.

Mapping Meaning: The Epidauria Procession

Given this historical context, I want to return briefly to Asklepios' arrival, to explore how his path into the city, as recorded on the Telemachos monument, could have been understood as articulating relations between Epidauros and Athens in the first years of the peace. This path would almost certainly have been repeated year after year in the Epidauria procession.

Admittedly, this is a dangerous exercise. As Denis Feeney has cautioned, rituals do not themselves say anything; rather, we make them say things, and so I am guilty of forcing the Epidauria's procession not only to speak but to say something that is quite possibly false.[37] Second, I am guilty of positing here a single voice when in fact there would have been multiple voices or readings— potentially as many as there were individuals to witness them. With these caveats in mind, I nevertheless venture to suggest one way in which the procession might have been interpreted.

The Telemachos monument, as we have seen, records several stops made by the god on his initial entry into Athens. His path began in Piraeus. As others have noted, the plague, too, entered Athens via Piraeus (Thucy. 2.48.2); thus, it was fitting that some ten years after the plague first struck, a famous healing god reached Athens through this same port, boding a new period of health for the city.[38]

It is also likely, given the involvement of *phrouroi* in the Epidauria and of the prominent role the Eleusinians played in Asklepios' arrival, that officials from the cults of both Asklepios at Epidauros and Demeter at Eleusis were present in Piraeus to escort the god to Athens. The procession thus prefigured from the outset the dual citizenship of the god, his ties both to his homeland, Epidauros, and now also to Athens. Significant in this regard is the fact that Asklepios arrived just as the annual military campaigning season was coming to a close (early October), and thus at a time when Athens was turning from warfare to more peaceful pursuits.

The new port of Piraeus, as opposed to the older port of Phaleron, marked the new national boundary. Piraeus' importance to Athenian naval supremacy and to control over the Delian League and eventually Athenian empire almost certainly nuanced the passage of Asklepios into Athens.[39] The emphasis on national boundaries also suggests the integration of a foreign power; much as other gods, like Thracian Bendis, would do, Asklepios traversed the watery border into Attica as a foreigner. The sea itself provided a potential allusion to yet another outsider welcomed into the Athenian pantheon: Poseidon. Poseidon lost the contest for control of Athens when his salty element failed to win as much favor among the citizens as Athena's olive, but he was nonetheless welcomed and integrated into the city, even onto the Acropolis.

After setting out from Piraeus, the procession headed towards Athens. Its centripetal motion drew Epidaurian Asklepios into the heart of the state and thereby brought the periphery (Epidauros) to the center of Athenian empire.[40] The most direct path for the procession would have been within the long walls, with entry through one of the southeastern gates. But, given the steep incline of this route, the procession may have traveled instead a road north of the walls where it would have joined the Sacred Way and entered the city via the Dipylon Gate. If so, it picked up the routes of several major festival processions, including those of the Panathenaia; of the initial procession of the City Dionysia, which reenacted the arrival of Dionysos from Eleutherai; and of that over which the sacred objects (the "holy things") were brought to Athens from Eleusis in preparation for the Mysteries. All of these processions, centripetal in motion like that of the Epidauria, marked the accession by Athens of border territories: of Eleutherai and Eleusis on the borders of Attica, and of the states that formed the borders of Athens' empire.[41]

Once inside the city, the procession moved towards the Eleusinion. The god entered this sanctuary just several days after the procession from Eleusis deposited the sacred objects there, so both the Epidauria and the Mysteries utilized the Eleusinion within a very brief period of time. Moreover, the primary responsibility for transporting the sacred objects to the Eleusinion rested with the Eumolpid family, descendants of Eumolpos, famous for having launched an attack against Athens at the time of King Erechtheus.[42] The Eumolpid attack resulted in the Athenian annexation of Eleusis, but only after much bloodshed. The Eleusinion marked the grave of Ismaros, Eumolpos' son and the one said by some sources to have led the attack against Athens. The entry of Eumolpos' descendants into the Eleusinion during the Mysteries may thus have symbolized the assimilation of this one-time Athenian enemy into the heart of the state; the invading enemy had become an ally of Athens.[43] Even the name of the sanctuary at which these events took place, the "Eleusinion," calls attention to the assimilation of Eleusis into Attica. In much the same way Epidaurian Asklepios, a representative of Athens' recent Peloponnesian enemy, followed Eumolpos' invasive route when he entered the Eleusinion only days later, during the "Epidauria," to be assimilated into Athens and Athenian empire.

The procession that accompanied Asklepios in 420 ended at the Eleusinion, where Asklepios' original journey initially stopped, but in subsequent years the procession must have continued on to the south slope of the Acropolis, where Asklepios had taken up residence by 419. According to the Telemachos monument, he was conveyed there via a *harma*, a kind of chariot having numerous associations with Athena (SEG 25.226, lines 14–15). Ancient sources attribute the chariot's invention to Athena, while others ascribe it to her foster son Erichthonios at the first celebration of the Panathenaia. Chariots played a major role in the Panathenaic games: in apobatic events, armed contestants jumped off and onto moving cars, while two- and four-horse chariot races (the latter vehicle being a *harma*) were also featured in the games. Chariots also stood to either side of Athena and Poseidon in the west pediment of the Parthenon, and apobatai with their four-horse chariots appear on the north and south sections of the Parthenon's frieze.[44] Another fifth-century tradition further reinforced the association between Athena and her chariot. According to Herodotus, when Peisistratos attempted to seize power a second time in Athens, he dressed a very tall woman named Phye in a suit of armor to look like Athena and rode into Athens on a *harma* next to the "goddess." Heralds ran ahead telling the Athenians that Athena herself was bringing Peisistratos back to her own citadel (Hdt. 1.60). Regarding Asklepios' arrival, it therefore seems that Athena, intent on extending an especially warm welcome to the god, sent her own special vehicle to escort him to his new sanctuary.[45]

The presence of a chariot or any other wheeled vehicle in the procession implies that the Epidauria continued east from the Eleusinion along the Street of the Tripods, the easiest path for wheeled vehicles heading to the south slope. After skirting the east end of the Acropolis, the procession would have ascended the south slope somewhere near the sanctuary of Dionysos.[46] The route thus followed that of the City Dionysia and brought Asklepios to his own precinct just next to that of Dionysos Eleuthereus, another relative newcomer to the Athenian pantheon. His arrival dates probably to the annexation of Eleutherai in the middle or late sixth century.[47]

The terminus of the Epidauria procession was almost certainly the Asklepieion, just below the Parthenon. Traveling the last leg of this procession on Athena's *harma*, Asklepios concluded his journey from Epidauros to Athens, a journey that symbolized his transition from being only Epidauros' god to being also an Athenian. The procession may have indicated to some that Athena and Asklepios had become neighbors and friends; consequently Epidauros and Athens were also friends and allies. As Numa Fustel de Coulanges long ago observed, "If [the ancients] could imagine that the protecting deities of two cities had some motive for becoming allies, this was reason enough why the two cities should become so."[48] But Athena was also patron of Athenian empire, and Epidauros had been subsumed symbolically into that empire. The topography of the Acropolis indicated a clear hierarchy: Asklepios' sanctuary lay below Athena's home on the summit. The two gods may have become friends, but they were not equals. Asklepios' presence in the Mysteries and Dionysia reinforced this ambiguity; Asklepios' participation in these spectacles and celebrations of Athenian empire implied his support of it. Thus, the procession of the

Epidauria could readily be perceived as articulating several messages at once: Asklepios was a favored member of the Athenian pantheon, but as such he was expected to defend Athens and its empire against, one would presume, even his homeland, Epidauros.[49]

Jonathan Hall has proposed that "the function of the hero is not so much to serve as an exclusive and static emblem of a city's distinctive identity, but to articulate the dynamic relationships that might exist between several cities." In this case we might easily substitute "god" for "hero," inasmuch as the deified Asklepios expressed just such a dynamic relationship between Epidauros and Athens.[50] Many aspects of Athens' reception of Epidaurian Asklepios suggest that the importation was an attempt to bring Epidauros under Athenian control. Prime among these was his integration into the Acropolis and the festivals of Dionysos Eleuthereus and Eleusinian Demeter. These places and rituals speak eloquently of the relations between cities and territories encompassed in the organization of Athenian empire, and of the diplomacy and alliances that contributed to its construction. Asklepios' importation came as the result of a host of factors, some of which are apparent to us (such as the lingering effects of plague and war) and others of which remain opaque, but the evidence gathered here suggests strongly that the god came in part to forge an alliance between Athens and a city critical to the preservation of Athenian empire.

Conclusions

Bonus intra, melior exi.
Enter a good person, leave a better one.

> *Inscription from the Asklepieion at*
> *Lambaesis, in Africa (CIL VIII.1.2584)*

The ongoing and far-reaching popularity of Asklepios' cult is firmly rooted in the fifth-century period of its development. At this time the cult achieved panhellenic fame and began its eventual spread across the Mediterranean. Whatever the additional reasons, local or translocal, that would attract individuals and communities to the god over time, it seems impossible that the cult would have taken such terrific hold without both the close ties to medicine and the relevance to politics that attached to the cult already in the fifth century BC.

The first of these two factors relates to the growing professionalization of medicine: namely, the decision of doctors, as attested in medical treatises, to refuse difficult cases in an effort to protect their credibility. As doctors were refusing to treat certain fatal and chronic conditions, individuals suffering many of the same chronic ailments sought help from the doctor-god, Asklepios. This factor in no way denies the effects of disruptions like war and plague on the popularity of the cult; rather, it affirms them while at the same time identifying a corresponding need for another healthcare alternative.

As medicine became a more widely accepted form of healing over time, the cult continued to grow. That the cult's appeal beyond the fifth century remained dependent in part upon the popularity of medicine is suggested in two ways. In cities with large medical centers, like Kos and Pergamon, the cult flourished. Conversely, in Republican Italy, where tradition holds that Greek medicine was accepted only with reluctance (Pliny NH 29.11–16), the cult enjoyed a much more limited following than in Greece.[1] Even after the cult's introduction to Rome at the start of the third century BC, few new sanctuaries of Asklepios (Aesculapius there) were established within Italy.[2]

The cult's success in curing chronically ill persons whom doctors could not or would not treat, when added to all of the other disruptions to individuals and the state traditionally adduced by scholars to account for Asklepios' appeal, goes a long way toward explaining both the increased number of visitors to sanctuaries of Asklepios and the popular demand for new sanctuaries in the fifth century. But, even when combined, these reasons alone are insufficient to account for the establishment of each new sanctuary, as is indicated by the importation of the cult to Athens in 420 BC. Here Asklepios' reception on the Acropolis slopes and the integration of his festivals into the City Dionysia and Eleusinian Mysteries all demonstrate a clear civic interest in the cult.

While the healing benefits of Asklepios surely contributed to Athens' interest in him, civic policy proves to have been another major factor. In the context of the Peloponnesian War, the importation of Epidauros' most famous god presented a convenient step toward bringing Epidauros under Athenian control, a goal expressed by Athens repeatedly in the 420s in its attempts to take Epidauros by force. It would thus seem that Epidaurian Asklepios, like Eleusinian Demeter, Dionysos Eleuthereus, Brauronian Artemis, and Thracian Bendis, was adopted and his cult adapted by Athens to advance its foreign policy, especially in regard to the acquisition of new territory. And so we must now recognize that Asklepios' appeal, in some instances at least, derived from concern over the body politic and not just over the individual bodies of a town.[3]

This was the case as well at Rome in the third century, as I have argued elsewhere, and is likely to be true also of the cult's development in places such as Kos and Pergamon, both with exceptionally large and popular cults of Asklepios and ties to powerful rulers (especially at Pergamon).[4] Here, too, locally and temporally specific factors should be considered when accounting for the cult's appeal. Nor must a relative paucity of evidence in comparison to Classical Athens necessarily stand in the way of studying the cult in other cities. Even in the case of Rome, where evidence from the Middle Republic is scant, sources can be used in innovative ways. As Peter Wiseman has stated regarding his own study of the development of the Remus myth, "It is true that the evidence for the period we are concerned with is desperately inadequate; but all that means is that hypotheses have to be carefully argued, and conclusions must be recognised as being necessarily provisional. What matters for the Remus myth is to recognise that explanation is needed."[5] The same is true for Asklepios.

Moreover, regarding cult transfer narratives, the Telemachos monument is instructive: we cannot assume that the Athenian cult was a "private" foundation just because a monument associates a particular individual with early events in its history. Similarly, other transfer narratives for Asklepios' cult that privilege individuals should not necessarily be taken as proof of "private" cult foundations.

This study began by questioning the application to the ancient world of dichotomies like public versus private, church versus state, and rational versus irrational. The model for Asklepios' cult advanced here disrupts these dichotomies; the cult is as much public as private, as appealing to the needs of the state as to the needs of individuals, and as rational as Greek medicine. These observations highlight the impossibility of distinguishing "religion" from the rest of ancient culture, even from aspects we now label "science," "medicine," or "politics." As Hugh Bowden has discussed, it is perhaps startling to realize that fifth-century Athens, the ideal to which modern democracies trace their roots, based its policies on the will of the divine, a practice more commonly associated in today's world with fundamentalist regimes whose obedience to the divine now evokes terror in democratic societies. To cast the image less starkly in terms of a model developed by Bruce Lincoln, Athens and other Greek states, regardless of their form of government, were maximalist rather than minimalist societies when it came to the gods.[6] For these Greeks, the gods were central to and took active part in the functioning of the state.

As to medicine, doctors, far from being opposed to Asklepios' cult, adopted Asklepios as their patron and served as his priests. Their understanding of the human body did not oppose belief in the divine per se; rather, it opposed the belief that the gods cause illness. And, while worship of the gods was not therefore a primary means of curing the body, the gods could assist in the healing process, particularly of cases beyond the capability of medicine. Perhaps the irony lies, then, not so much in the juncture of medicine and cult in antiquity but in the persistent use of the staff and serpent of Asklepios today by a medical profession deemed separate from religion.

But is the current practice of medicine really so separate from religion? It is certainly not separable from rituals. Visiting a Western physician today, particularly in the United States, is in some striking ways similar to the experience of an ancient visitor to an Asklepieion. Just as one in antiquity had to travel to Asklepios' sanctuary for healing (physicians from antiquity to the early twentieth century, by contrast, more typically made house calls), today we go to the doctor's office, clinic, or hospital, where we undergo certain preliminary rituals upon entering the facility, such as talking to a receptionist to whom we hand insurance cards and the like. Then we sit and wait, sometimes for long periods, to see an attendant—often a nurse, attired in identifying clothing, so we know that he or she is an authority—who checks our vital signs and then ushers us into a smaller, more private room, where we strip off our clothes and don the same robe as every other patient. We wait again, this time in anticipation of the physician. As we wait, we gaze at the medical diplomas on the wall and the array of instruments that might be sitting on counters, all meant to assure us of the healer's authority, competence, and training—not so different from the effect of the iamata, anatomical votives, and other dedications displayed conspicuously at Asklepieia. Finally, the epiphany: the physician enters, sporting a white lab coat, stethoscope wound round the neck, much like Asklepios who invariably appears in his himation (long cloak), walking staff at hand.

The examination might take only a fraction of the time of these preliminaries, but the preliminaries themselves—whatever their practical function—can also have a very real physical as well as emotional effect on the patient and thus on the healing process. Some aspects of the experience, such as the unusual, intimidating environment (the modern, sterile, bright clinic, hospital, or doctor's office; the ancient sanctuary with its sacred animals) in which people sick with various illnesses come and go and the patient is treated apart from family and friends, may increase patient anxiety. Doctors, for instance, report that patient blood pressures recorded in their offices are often higher than normal, and a healing inscription from Epidauros describes a mute girl who is suddenly able to yell for her parents when frightened by a snake moving about the Asklepieion.[7]

Other aspects of these experiences, such as the diplomas and healing inscriptions, have the potential to generate a greater sense of confidence in the healer and the techniques and treatments. The "placebo effect" of therapeutic measures is much debated in the scientific community and largely speculative due to the difficulty of subjecting it to empirical analysis; but we may well be mistaken to discount entirely the importance of pre-examination rituals to patient recovery, given their prominence in encounters both with Asklepios in antiquity and with physicians today.[8] I therefore remain enamored of the idea that, in addition to the many salutary benefits of fresh water, rest, exercise, and the like afforded by Asklepieia, the cumulative result of all the preliminary rites at these sanctuaries inspired greater faith in Asklepios, which in turn had a positive effect on the efficacy of his cures.

This is not to say that we in the twenty-first century perceive medicine as miracle and physicians as divine. However, in many of these ritual aspects, the similarities between visiting Asklepios and visiting our typical doctor are strong. So perhaps it is entirely fitting after all that Asklepios, albeit in a more secularized and depoliticized guise, continues his august watch over the medical community some twenty-five hundred years after the initial surge in his cult's popularity.

Introduction

1. Asklepios' myth is discussed in more detail in Chapter 3 below. For ancient sources on Asklepios, see Edelstein and Edelstein 1945, esp. vol. 1, Testimonies 1–122, and for further discussion, vol. 2, 22–53.

2. Excavation of Asklepios' sanctuaries at Athens and Epidauros began in the 1870s and 1880s, respectively. For the excavation history of Asklepieia in Greece, see the following, which include discussion and bibliography arranged by sanctuary: Semeria 1986; Melfi 2003 (now superseded by Melfi 2007, although the earlier work includes many sanctuaries not covered in the latter); Riethmüller 2005, vol. 2. Riethmüller also catalogues evidence for cults of Asklepios outside Greece. For a survey of scholarship on Asklepios and his cult, see Wickkiser 2003, 2–6; Riethmüller 2005, vol. 1, 21–30.

3. Edelstein and Edelstein 1945, vol. 1, p. xxiii–xxiv: "One thing, however, must be emphasized: the material here taken into consideration is restricted to the written evidence. . . . The study of the monuments requires an approach very different from that to be applied to the study of the literary remains; to combine both methods within the compass of one inquiry seemed impossible." On this and other limitations of Edelstein and Edelstein 1945, see the judicious assessment by Gary Ferngren in his new introduction to the 1998 edition of their work. Ferngren (xiii–xiv) explains that Sigerist was director of the Institute for the History of Medicine at Johns Hopkins University in Baltimore and had invited Ludwig to join his staff. Ludwig, forced out of his native Germany by the Nazi regime, taught at Hopkins from 1934 into 1947.

4. Riethmüller 2005; Melfi 2003 and 2007.

5. E.g., Edelstein and Edelstein (1945, vol. 2, 154) speak of the "irrational" element in Asklepios' cures.

6. On the nature of Frazer's project and how it developed over time, see J.Z. Smith 1978, 208–239; Fraser 1990; Beard 1992. Kee 1983 discusses Frazer's work in relation to other major studies in the history of religion.

7. Dodds 1951, 193. The model of a primitive medicine that relies heavily on magic and religion in contrast to a modern medicine that utilizes rational techniques with little magico-religious influence also dominated anthropological studies of health in the first

half of the twentieth century, as apparent in the works of W.H.R. Rivers and Erwin Ackerknecht (e.g., Rivers 1924; Ackerknecht 1946).

8. Dodds 1977, 97; also 97–111 passim.

9. King 2006, 248.

10. E.g., Behr 1968, 36; Kee 1982, 124–125, 134–136; Temkin 1991, 171–196; Cotter 1999; Gorrini 2005.

11. E.g., Edelstein and Edelstein 1945, vol. 2, 154. On the use of dreams in ancient medical prognosis as being a rational practice, see van der Eijk 2004, with references. On dreams in Greco-Roman medicine, see also Oberhelman 1993.

12. Harrison 2006, 136. Lloyd 1979, 49; see also Lloyd 1970, 1979, 1983, 1987, and 2003. The impact of Lloyd's arguments is increasingly evident in studies of other ancient healing cults, such as C.M.C. Green's discussion of the cult of Diana at Aricia (2007, esp. 235–279).

13. Edelstein and Edelstein 1945, vol. 2, 132–138.

14. Edelstein and Edelstein 1945, vol. 2, 176.

15. E.g., Ar. Pl. 653f.; *I.Perg.* III 161, a second-century AD law from the sanctuary of Asklepios at Pergamon that describes the remuneration required for incubation. On this inscription, see also Lupu 2005, 61–63. Comparison of Asklepios to Christ was criticized by Vlastos (1949). For the role of healing and charity in early Christianity, see Ferngren 1992.

16. The most famous example of *evocatio* is the transferal of Juno from Etruscan Veii to Rome, recorded by Livy 5.21.1–7. On *evocatio*, see Beard et al. 1998, 34–35, with n. 97 for bibliography.

17. J.K. Davies in *CAH²*, vol. 4, p. 372; Garland 1992, 130. Also Hölscher 1991, 376: "The most important new sanctuary [of the late Classical period] was not dedicated to the deity of a political state cult but to Asclepius, the god of healing."

18. E.g., J.Z. Smith 2004, 179–196; Masuzawa 2005, esp. 37–71. Recent studies of colonialism have directed more attention to this topic: e.g., Chidester 1996, esp. 1–29 (southern Africa); Lopez 1998, esp. 156–180 (Tibet). Others, however, maintain the view that Greeks and Romans conceptualized religion as a distinct cognitive domain; e.g., Woolf 1997. On the difficulty of defining and delimiting religion in contemporary society, see Asad 1993, 27–54, originally published in *Man* 18 (1983) 237–259; also Lincoln 2003, with particular reference to the impact of events of September 11, 2001. My thanks to Brent Nongbri for many enlightening discussions on this topic. Asklepios' apparent separation from politics may also derive in part from his being a doctor, a profession generally idealized in the modern world as apolitical or at least nonpartisan.

19. J.P. Davies 2004, 7, following Feeney 1998, 12–13. Similarly, Boedeker (2007, 46) begins her chapter on Athenian religion in the *Cambridge Companion to the Age of Pericles* with what is becoming a standard disclaimer about the lack of a Greek term corresponding to our word "religion," and then goes on to state that "acts performed in recognition of unseen powers intermingled constantly with other aspects of daily life, rather than defining a discrete area of human activity." Also Connelly 2007, esp. 4–6, although Connelly, like many scholars, continues to employ these categories after arguing that they did not exist in antiquity (e.g., "Even when [Greek] women are recognized as central players in the *religious sphere* . . ." 276, emphasis added). It is becoming increasingly common to see schol-

ars describing "religion" as "embedded" in ancient Greek and Roman culture. On the prevalence of and problems inherent in this terminology, see Nongbri 2008.

20. Bowden 2005, 2. Bowden has been criticized for seeing too much similarity between Athenian democracy and fundamentalist societies in which the state functions to enact divine will; see, e.g., the review by Timothy Howe in *Bryn Mawr Classical Review* 2006.7.13.

21. Aleshire 1989, 14–15. For other descriptions of the Athenian cult as private, see Garland 1992, 128–130; Aleshire 1994; Parker 1996, 180–181; Stafford 2000, 155, with n. 33; also Dignas 2007, 175–176, who posits a general pattern of transformation from private foundation to public cult in many sanctuaries of Asklepios, while also recognizing that the evidence does not neatly fit such a strict dichotomy.

22. Aleshire 1989, 14, n. 5.

23. Parker 1996, 6. Also Sourvinou-Inwood 1988, esp. 270–273; Sourvinou-Inwood 1990; Bruit Zaidman and Schmitt Pantel 1992, 63; Parker 1996, 5–6. Bruit Zaidman and Schmitt Pantel write that the label "domestic" or "family" religion "is inadequate, because the rituals in question are as much civic as domestic, and the cleavage familiar today between private and public life has hardly any meaning in a context where matrimonial and funerary rituals were a matter of concern to the community at large, not just the few individuals immediately involved."

24. Sourvinou-Inwood 1990, 297. In another context, she remarks, "All cult acts, including those which some modern commentators are inclined to think of as 'private,' are (religiously) dependent on the polis" (Sourvinou-Inwood 1988, 270). For an opposing view, see J.K. Davies in *CAH*², vol. 4, 370.

25. E.g., IG I³ 7, 14, 34, 35, 38, 133, 136, 138. See Garland 1992, 99–115 for discussion of these decrees and for the increasing involvement of the demos in Athenian religion.

26. Egretes, known from a single inscription of 306/5 BC found at the base of the Hill of the Nymphs, had his own sanctuary in which he was worshipped by a group of individuals called *orgeones*. On Egretes, see Ferguson 1944, 79–81; Parker 1996, 109–111. Parker questions the traditional assumption that groups of *orgeones* be perceived as private associations only with no public dimension. On *orgeones*, see also Ferguson 1944; Kearns 1989, 73–77.

27. War and plague: Avalos 1999, 50–51; mounting tension and insecurity during the war: Hölscher 1991; rising acceptance of "the irrational": Dodds 1951; craving for more personal attention from the gods: Edelstein and Edelstein 1945, vol. 2, 111–118; Mitropoulou 1975, 11; Amundsen and Ferngren 1982, 77.

28. The work of Catherine Bell, esp. Bell 1992 and 1997, has been particularly influential for my analysis.

One • From Practice to Profession

1. In the *Odyssey*, for example, Odysseus' cousins, who are not healers by trade, adeptly heal his boar wound (*Od.* 19.447–462). The average person probably could not have named a particular individual as their teacher but would have acquired healing knowledge from various sources.

2. One of the best general, well-referenced discussions of ancient Greek healing practices is Majno 1975. Not only is it highly readable and accessible to those with little or no background on the subject, but it discusses healing practices of other ancient cultures. For a more detailed overview of medicine in ancient Greece and Rome, see Nutton 2004. On social aspects of ancient medicine, see also Nutton 1992, 1995a, 1995b, 1995c. On the use of drugs by healers, see Scarborough 1991. On ἰατρομάντεις, see Dodds 1951, 135–178.

3. The prayers of magicians were not very different from the prayers of the priests in terms of structure, content, and context, as Graf (1991) has shown. Moreover, Rufus of Ephesus (fr. 90) categorizes amulets among medical cures (possibly because they were thought to act by physical means, such as giving off aromas; cf. Galen, SMT [Kühn 11.859–860]), and Soranus of Ephesus says amulets should be used in certain cases because they can make patients more cheerful (Sor. Gyn. 3.42.3). See also Lloyd 1979, 42; Scarborough 1991, 159.

4. King 1998, 159, comments: "[The authors of the Hippocratic corpus] place what they do within the context of a divinely ordered universe but, although they are not opposed to religious systems of healing, they see no particular deity as being responsible for the cures they effect." I would extend that last clause to include not just deities but any other being, whether mortal or immortal.

5. One might use a phrase like "natural healing" instead of "medicine" to avoid the teleological connotations of the latter, but such a term presents its own problems. "Natural healing," for example, suggests that what Greek doctors practiced was opposed to "supernatural healing," which is misleading not least because many doctors believed nature itself to be divine. See also Chapter 2 below.

6. On spices in Linear B tablets, see Wylock 1972; Janko 1981; Shelmerdine 1985, 130; R. Arnott 1996, 267–268. On Bronze Age skeletal remains and medical instruments, see R. Arnott 1996, 266, 268–269; and 1999, 501–504. R. Arnott 1996, 269, notes that the burial of instruments along with the tomb's occupant indicates high social status of the deceased. On i-ja-te, see R. Arnott 1996, 266; and 2004, 157. Laskaris 1999, 1–2, emphasizes cross-cultural contacts of medical experts in the Bronze Age Aegean; also Laskaris 2002, 32–39.

7. On the nature of the Iliad plague, see Hankinson 1995, 27–29.

8. On the treatment of war wounds in antiquity as described by literary sources and as documented in the material record, see Salazar 2000.

9. Il. 5.902–904: "As when fig juice by its force congeals white milk while liquid and very quickly forms curdles for the one stirring, just as quickly did [Paieon] heal raging Ares." (ὡς δ' ὅτ ὀπὸς γάλα λευκὸν ἐπειγόμενος συνέπηξεν | ὑγρὸν ἐόν, μάλα δ' ὦκα περιτρέφεται κυκόωντι, | ὣς ἄρα καρπαλίμως ἰήσατο θοῦρον Ἄρηα.) Paieon also heals Hades using a poultice of drugs, Il. 5.401.

10. Remarkably, the healers who use both bandages (δῆσαν ἐπισταμένως) and incantations (ἐπαοιδῇ) to treat Odysseus' boar wound in the Odyssey are not called iatroi. On the infrequent use of incantations in medicine, see Chapter 2 below.

11. We cannot be sure the Greeks understood infection based on the treatments as they are recorded; Western medicine before Semmelweiss in the mid-nineteenth century seems not to have shown any regard for basic cleanliness, and it is not until Lister later in

the same century that doctors began routinely using antiseptics. Nevertheless, the possibility remains that they did, especially since there are allusions to internal medicine in early poetry, including Homer (e.g., *Od.* 4.230–231 on Egypt as a land yielding many drugs). For allusions to internal medicine in early poetry, see Dean-Jones 2003, 99–100.

12. Il. 11.514–515: ἰητρὸς γὰρ ἀνὴρ πολλῶν ἀντάξιος ἄλλων | ἰούς τ' ἐκτάμνειν ἐπί τ' ἤπια φάρμακα πάσσειν.

13. *Od.* 17.382–386: "For who himself approaches and calls in a stranger from another place, unless that man is a worker of the people—a prophet or healer of ills or crafter of wood, or a divine singer who gives delight by singing? For these men are famous across the boundless earth." (τίς γὰρ δὴ ξεῖνον καλεῖ ἄλλοθεν αὐτὸς ἐπελθὼν | ἄλλον γ', εἰ μὴ τῶν οἳ δημιοεργοὶ ἔασι; | μάντιν ἢ ἰητῆρα κακῶν ἢ τέκτονα δούρων, | ἢ καὶ θέσπιν ἀοιδόν, ὅ κεν τέρπησιν ἀείδων; | οὗτοι γὰρ κλητοί γε βροτῶν ἐπ' ἀπείρονα γαῖαν.)

14. Solon, quoted by Stob. 3.9.23 = IE² Fr. 13.57–62: ἄλλοι Παιῶνος πολυφαρμάκου ἔργον ἔχοντες | ἰητροί· καὶ τοῖς οὐδὲν ἔπεστι τέλος· | πολλάκι δ' ἐξ ὀλίγης ὀδύνης μέγα γίγνεται ἄλγος, κοὐκ ἄν τις λύσαιτ' ἤπια φάρμακα δούς· | τὸν δὲ κακαῖς νούσοισι κυκώμενον ἀργαλέαις τε | ἁψάμενος χειροῖν αἶψα τίθησ' ὑγιῆ.

15. See below on the development of internal medicine in the seventh century BC. Cupping instruments are attested by the late sixth century BC; see the discussion of the Basel relief below in this chapter.

16. In the Arktinos fragment, Machaon and Podaleirios seem to have been granted, not taught, healing skills. This difference between being granted and being taught is important to the concept of a *techne*, characterized as a rationally explicable skill transmitted through teaching rather than inspiration.

17. On the development of both and their mutual impact, see Lloyd 1979; Longrigg 1993. On the development of naturalistic explanation, see also Hankinson 1998a, esp. ch 1.

18. Sen. *Q Nat.* 3.14: "The following idea of Thales is foolish. For he says that the circle of the world sits supported by water and is borne along like a ship, and when it is said to shake, it rocks with the movement of the water. 'Thus it is no wonder that there is more than enough water to make the rivers flow since the whole circle is in water.'" (*Quae sequitur Thaletis inepta sententia est. Ait enim terrarum orbem aqua sustineri et uehi more nauigii, mobilitateque fluctuare tunc cum dicitur tremere; "non est ergo mirum si abundat umor ad flumina profundenda, cum in umore sit totus."*) Text is that of H.M. Hine (Teubner).

19. Aëtius 5.30.1 = DK 24B4: "[Alcmaeon] says that the equality of the powers—wet and dry, hot and cold, bitter and sweet, and the rest—preserves health, and that any one of them gaining control over the others is the cause of illness." (ἔφη τῆς μὲν ὑγιείας εἶναι συνεκτικὴν τὴν ἰσονομίαν τῶν δυνάμεων ὑγροῦ ξηροῦ θερμοῦ πικροῦ γλυκέος καὶ τῶν λοιπῶν, τὴν δ' ἐν αὐτοῖς μοναρχίαν νόσου παρασκευαστικὴν εἶναι.) This theory bears a strong resemblance to that of the slightly earlier Anaximander of Miletos, who believed that the cosmos was a balance between opposites (Simplicius *In physica* 24.13 = DK 12B1). Metaphors of justice are important in the writings of both: See Longrigg 1993, esp. 47–81.

20. For the brain as the seat of the intellect: Aëtius 5.17.3 = DK 24A13; for semen as the substance of the brain: Aëtius 5.3.3 = DK 24A13. Longrigg 1993, 54–57, provides a useful table comparing Alcmaeon's queries into the physiology of the body with those of other natural philosophers.

21. Theophr. *Fragment on Sensation*, 25–26 = DK 24A5.

22. I owe this observation to Lesley Dean-Jones.

23. The tradition of the "Hippocratic" treatises is discussed in more detail below. Among the treatises to which scholars assign an early date are *Diseases II*, ca. 450 (Jouanna 1999); *Gynecology*, ca. 480 BC (Grensemann 1987); *Airs, Waters, Places*, pre-Herodotus (Thomas 1993); *Places in Man* (Craik 1998).

24. Hankinson (1991, 87) succinctly addresses the later distinction of Kos and Knidos, as well as cities in southern Italy (like Croton), as centers of medical training. He lists relevant bibliography, including especially Thivel 1981.

25. He also treats Darius' wife Atossa for an abscess on her breast (Hdt. 3.133).

26. On public doctors in ancient Greece, see Cohn-Haft 1956; Pleket 1983. What exactly a public doctor was and did is open to debate, but in Athens by the fifth century BC the position was certainly an elected one. Cohn-Haft proposes that the demos secured a public doctor to ensure the services of at least one skilled healer during a time when demand for doctors outweighed their supply. Jouanna (1999, 77–78) instead attributes the office to a desire to secure the services of a competent doctor in particular.

27. Antikenmuseum, Basel, inv. no. BS 236. The dating is contested: Berger (1970, 30–33) dates it to ca. 480 BC on stylistic grounds, while Nutton (1992, 20) maintains a sixth-century date.

28. A famous example is the second-century AD tombstone of the Athenian doctor Jason (British Museum, inv. no. GR 1865.1–1.3), well illustrated in Berger 1970, 78, fig. 99; Nutton 2004, fig. 6.1; the inscription: IG II² 4513.

29. For illustrations and discussion of cupping instruments, see Krug 1985, 96–97.

30. Dean-Jones (2003, 116–118) argues against the generally held view that physicians were itinerant. The walking staff of physicians then may have more to do with the traditional iconography of Asklepios and his mythology than with an assumed itinerancy of individual physicians.

31. National Archaeological Museum, Athens, inv. no. 93; IG I³ 1393 = Friedländer and Hoffleit 1948, 16 no. 8. The lettering on the disk is Attic, although the original provenance of the object is unknown; see Jeffrey 1962, 147, no. 66; Berger 1970, 155–158; Samama 2003, no. 001. It is also illustrated and discussed in Marshall 1909, 154; Berger 1970, 157. On the function of the disk, see Marshall 1909, 154. It is striking that the word *sophia* appears in the inscription instead of *techne*, which may reflect the early date of the monument. For other epigraphic sources related to Greek medicine, see Samama 2003.

32. As Pleket (1995) has cautioned, many doctors never attained high social status. The examples discussed here, however, demonstrate that some clearly could and did attain a comfortable level of status and wealth.

33. Louvre, inv. no. CA 2183.

34. Ar. Pl. 407–408: Τίς δῆτ' ἰατρός ἐστι νῦν ἐν τῇ πόλει; / Οὔτε γὰρ ὁ μισθὸς οὐδὲν· ἔστ' οὔθ' ἡ τέχνη.Text is that of F.W. Hall and W.M. Geldart (Oxford Classical Texts). On doctors in Greek comedy, see Alfageme 1995.

35. On the competitive nature of the posts, see Pl. *Grg.* 456b–c, where Gorgias contends that a sophist, by reason of his ability to speak and thus persuade the assembly, could easily win the position any day and anywhere over a qualified doctor.

36. See Longrigg 1993.

37. Jouanna 1999, 6.

38. The dissemination of medical treatises by Hippocrates may have facilitated Athenian awareness of him. For the general impact on Greek medicine of the spread of medical texts in the fifth and fourth centuries BC, see Dean-Jones 2003.

39. Scrib.Larg. Comp. 5: *Conditor nostrae professionis*; Sen. Ep. 95.20: *maximus ille medicorum et huius scientiae conditor*; Celsus *De med.* 1.praef.8: *Hippocrates Cous, primus ex omnibus memoria dignus . . . uir et arte et facundia insignis*. On Galen's admiration for Hippocrates, see W.D. Smith 1979, 61–176; Temkin 1991, 47–50; King 2006, 257–258 (and *passim* on the gradual shift in antiquity from viewing Hippocrates as a great physician to being the founder, and later also father, of medicine; also King 2002).

40. The ending -*ike* is an adjective-producing suffix, and *iatrike* is thus originally an adjectival form related to *iatros*. *Iatrike* probably began as modifying the word *techne*; see Chantraine 1956, 115, 129–130.

41. Aristophanes, poking fun not only at the wealth of new *technai*, but also acknowledging the place of *iatrike* in the late fifth century BC, coins the word ἰατροτέχνη in the *Clouds*, produced in 423 (*Nub.* 332). It is not surprising that the chorus of Clouds are thought to nourish not only *iatrotechne* but also sophists, particularly those from Thurii in southern Italy (*Nub.* 331–334), since southern Italy was the home of both doctors (Democedes, Alcmaeon, etc.) and sophists (e.g., Gorgias) vital to the development of *rhetorike*. *Techne*, or skill, has a range of meanings from Homer on, including the sometimes-negative connotations of cunning and trickery. Hankinson (1991, 82–83) provides a useful summary of its range of meanings over time; for a more detailed discussion, see Isnardi Parente 1966.

42. *De arte* 1 = 6.2 L.: "There are some who have made a *techne* out of villifying the *technai*." (Εἰσί τινες οἳ τέχνην πεποίηνται τὸ τὰς τέχνας αἰσχροεπεῖν.) The author concludes his introduction, however, by stating that he will respond in particular to attacks against *iatrike*.

43. On the development of rhetoric as a *techne*, see Kennedy 1963; Cole 1991.

44. *Iatrike* is also important as an example of a *techne* in Plato's *Ion* (537–540), and is a paradigm *techne* for Plato (e.g., *Prt.*) and Aristotle.

45. On the dating of the treatise, see Jouanna 1990, 81–85; Hankinson 1992, 55 n. 2; Dunn 2005, esp. 49–50.

46. On the linguistic development of "iatrike" and other ancient Greek medical vocabulary, see van Brock 1961, 5. On the evolution of the -*ikos* ending, see Chantraine 1956, 97–171. A work of Empedocles is referred to by various ancient sources as Ἰατρικὸς λόγος and Περὶ ἰατρικῆς (Diog. 8.77 = DK 31A1; Pliny NH 29.1.5 = DK 31A3). If the work was so named by Empedocles (ca. 492–432 BC), then the term may have been in use earlier in the fifth century than Herodotus. The term also appears in certain medical treatises that may well predate Herodotus, but by how much is a matter of speculation. On the occurrence of "iatrike" in the medical treatises and on the problems of dating these treatises, see below in this chapter.

47. The Hippocratic corpus contains more than sixty treatises varying in style, vocabulary, and even theory. On its editing by Alexandrian scholars, see Jouanna 1999, 348–353. Littré's edition, dating 1839–1861 and abbreviated as "L." in my quotations of the Hippocratic texts, is the most recent complete edition. Jouanna 1999, App. 3, provides

a catalogue of the treatises in alphabetical order by title, with a summary of their contents and their probable dates. While not all scholars agree with Jouanna's dates (in fact, it is hard to find any two scholars who agree about the dating of all of the treatises in the corpus), the catalogue is useful because it includes his dating criteria. The first scholar known to have tackled the issue of authenticity in the Hippocratic corpus is Erotian in the first century AD. For a summary of the ancient and modern debates concerning Hippocratic authorship, see W.D. Smith 1979, esp. 14–43; Jouanna 1999, 58–65.

48. The question of the target audiences of individual Hippocratic treatises has recently attracted attention; see, e.g., Thomas 1993; Laskaris 2002, 73–124. It is clear that some of the treatises speak to an audience already practicing iatrikē (e.g., Airs, Waters, Places; Nature of Man), while others speak to those with some knowledge in iatrikē but who are not necessarily iatroi (e.g., On the Art). Dean-Jones 2002 argues that most of the treatises were meant as teaching texts.

49. Aer. 1 = 2.12 L.: Ἰητρικὴν ὅστις βούλεται ὀρθῶς ζητεῖν, τάδε χρὴ ποιεῖν. New editions of the text have been produced by Diller (1970) and Jouanna (1996).

50. Morb.Sacr. 1, 3 = 6.354, 366 L.: Ἐμοὶ δὲ δοκέουσιν οἱ πρῶτοι τοῦτο τὸ νόσημα ἱερώσαντες τοιοῦτοι εἶναι ἄνθρωποι οἷοι καὶ νῦν εἰσι μάγοι τε καὶ καθάρται καὶ ἀγύρται καὶ ἀλαζόνες, οὗτοι δὲ καὶ προσποιέονται σφόδρα θεοσεβέες εἶναι καὶ πλέον τι εἰδέναι. Οὗτοι τοίνυν παραμπεχόμενοι καὶ προβαλλόμενοι τὸ θεῖον τῆς ἀμηχανίης τοῦ μὴ ἔχειν ὅ τι προσενέγκοντες ὠφελήσουσιν, καὶ ὡς μὴ κατάδηλοι ἔωσιν οὐδὲν ἐπιστάμενοι, ἱερὸν ἐνόμισαν τοῦτο τὸ πάθος εἶναι . . . Ἀλλὰ γὰρ αἴτιος ὁ ἐγκέφαλος τούτου τοῦ πάθεος, ὥσπερ καὶ τῶν ἄλλων νουσημάτων τῶν μεγίστων. Jouanna (2003) has published a new edition of the text with commentary.

51. De arte 3 = 6.4 L.: Περὶ δὲ ἰητρικῆς, ἐς ταύτην γὰρ ὁ λόγος, ταύτης οὖν τὴν ἀπόδειξιν ποιήσομαι, καὶ πρῶτόν γε διοριεῦμαι ὃ νομίζω ἰητρικὴν εἶναι. Some scholars have argued that the rhetorical style of the treatise suggests its author was a sophist; for discussion and bibliography, see Mann 2005, 1–22. Mann proposes that the author may be Antiphon. Jouanna (1988) has published a new edition of the text with commentary.

52. Prog. 1 = 2.110 L.: "For it is impossible to make healthy all who are sick." (Ὑγιέας μὲν γὰρ ποιεῖν ἅπαντας τοὺς νοσέοντας ἀδύνατον.) According to Jouanna (1999, App. 3.48), ancient critics unanimously attributed this treatise to Hippocrates; it may thus belong to the second half of the fifth century.

53. Prorrh. II 8 = 9.26 L.: "Concerning those suffering from gout, the following holds: all who are old or have concretions at their joints or live a sedentary life and are constipated, these are all incurable by human skill, as for as I know." Περὶ δὲ ποδαγρώντων τάδε· ὅσοι μὲν γέροντες ἢ περὶ τοῖσιν ἄρθροισιν ἐπιπωρώματα ἔχουσιν, ἢ τρόπον ἀταλαίπωρον ζῶσι κοιλίας ξηρὰς ἔχοντες, οὗτοι μὲν πάντες ἀδύνατοι ὑγιέες γίνεσθαι ἀνθρωπίνῃ τέχνῃ, ὅσον ἐγὼ οἶδα.) The cases of gout he considers incurable are those contracted by old people or those who have concretions at their joints or who do not exercise and suffer from constipation. Jouanna (1999, App. 3.50) dates the treatise to the second half of the fifth century BC. García Novo (1995) has followed others in arguing for a fourth-century date on the basis of style and language primarily, but her evidence could support an earlier date.

54. Morb.Sacr. 2 = 6.364 L.: "This disease seems to me no more divine than any others; rather, just like other diseases, it has a nature and cause that accounts for it; and it

seems to me no less curable than other diseases, unless so much time has passed and it has become so entrenched that it is already stronger than the remedies applied." (Τὸ δὲ νόσημα τοῦτο οὐδέν τί μοι δοκεῖ θειότερον εἶναι τῶν λοιπῶν, ἀλλὰ φύσιν μὲν ἔχει ἣν καὶ τὰ ἄλλα νοσήματα, καὶ πρόφασιν ὅθεν ἕκαστα γίνεται· καὶ ἰητὸν εἶναι, καὶ οὐδὲν ἧσσον ἑτέρων, ὅ τι ἂν μὴ ἤδη ὑπὸ χρόνου πολλοῦ καταβεβιασμένον ᾖ, ὥστε ἤδη εἶναι ἰσχυρότερον εἶναι τῶν φαρμάκων τῶν προσφερομένων.)

55. De arte 8 = 6.12–14 L.: Εἰ γάρ τις ἢ τέχνην ἐς ἃ μὴ τέχνη, ἢ φύσιν ἐς ἃ μὴ φύσις πέφυκεν, ἀξιώσειε δύνασθαι, ἀγνοεῖ ἄγνοιαν ἁρμόζουσαν μανίῃ μᾶλλον ἢ ἀμαθίῃ. Ὧν γὰρ ἐστιν ἡμῖν τοῖσί τε τῶν φυσίων τοῖσί τε τῶν τεχνέων ὀργάνοις ἐπικρατεῖν τουτῶν ἐστιν ἡμῖν δημιουργοῖς εἶναι, ἄλλων δὲ οὐκ ἔστιν. Note the echo of demioergos from the Odyssey.

56. De arte 8 = 6.14 L.: Παρακελευόμενοι δὲ ταῦτα ὑπὸ μὲν τῶν οὐνόματι ἰητρῶν θαυμά-ζονται, ὑπὸ δὲ τῶν καὶ τέχνῃ καταγελῶνται. Οὐ μὴν οὕτως ἀφρόνων οἱ ταύτης τῆς δημιουργίης ἔμπειροι οὔτε μωμητέων οὔτ' ἐπαινετέων δέονται· ἀλλὰ λελογισμένων πρὸς ὅ τι αἱ ἐργασίαι τῶν δημιουργῶν τελευτώμεναι πλήρεις εἰσί, καὶ ὅτευ ὑπολειπόμεναι ἐνδεεῖς, ἔτι τῶν ἐνδειῶν, ἅς τε τοῖς δημιουργεῦσιν ἀναθετέον ἅς τε τοῖς δημιουργεομένοισιν. Note again the echo of demioergos from the Odyssey.

57. The author begins his treatise by addressing the disparagement of the arts in general; only in Section 3 does he channel his arguments into a defense specifically of medicine.

58. De arte 3 = 6.4-6 L.: "First I will explain what I believe iatrike to be: it is releasing from illness all those who suffer, lessening of the severity of diseases, and not treating those who are overpowered by their illnesses, knowing that iatrike is not able to treat these things." Πρῶτόν γε διοριεῦμαι ὃ νομίζω ἰητρικὴν εἶναι· τὸ δὴ πάμπαν ἀπαλλάσσειν τῶν νοσεόντων τοὺς καμάτους καὶ τῶν νοσημάτων τὰς σφοδρότητας ἀμβλύνειν, καὶ τὸ μὴ ἐγχειρεῖν τοῖσι κεκρατημένοις ὑπὸ τῶν νοσημάτων, εἰδότας ὅτι ταῦτα οὐ δύναται ἰητρική.)

59. De arte 14 = 6.26 L.: "Both the present writings and the demonstrations of those who are knowledgeable of this techne make it clear that iatrike has in itself a rich store of arguments on its own behalf, and that it would be perfectly just in not treating difficult cases, or, if such cases are undertaken, would render their practitioners blameless." (Ὅτι μὲν οὖν καὶ λόγους ἐν ἑωυτῇ εὐπόρους ἐς τὰς ἐπικουρίας ἔχει ἡ ἰητρική, καὶ οὐκ εὐδι-ορθώτοισι δικαίως οὐκ ἂν ἐγχειροίη τῇσι νούσοισιν, ἢ ἐγχειρευμένας ἀναμαρτήτους ἂν παρέχοι, οἵ τε νῦν λεγόμενοι λόγοι δηλοῦσιν αἵ τε τῶν εἰδότων τὴν τέχνην ἐπιδείξιες.) The author now adds another clause to his argument: if doctors should undertake cases that are impossible to cure, they are not to be blamed if the afflicted person does not improve.

60. The citations are too numerous to list here, but they can be found in von Staden 1990; Prioreschi 1992; and Amundsen 1996, 30–49. Von Staden 1990 also includes a valuable discussion of the differences in vocabulary used to designate a case as "untreatable."

61. Morb. II 48 = 7.72 L.: Τοῦτον μὴ ἰᾶσθαι ὅταν οὕτως ἔχῃ. Jouanna (1999, App. 3.16) claims that the material contained in Diseases II is possibly mid-fifth century but that the treatise underwent several rewritings.

62. Morb. I 6 = 6.150 L.: "[The physician] acts properly in this way but improperly in the following: he behaves improperly . . . when he does not fully cure what can be cured,

and when he claims that he will fully cure what cannot be cured. (Ὀρθῶς δ᾿ ἐν αὐτῇ καὶ οὐκ ὀρθῶς τὰ τοιάδε· οὐκ ὀρθῶς μὲν ... τὰ δυνατὰ μὴ ἐξιᾶσθαι, καὶ τὰ ἀδύνατα φάναι ἐξιήσεσθαι.) Jouanna (1999, App. 3.15) dates the treatise to the 380s BC.

63. Wittern 1979; von Staden 1990. On the distinction between "supportive treatment" and treatment meant to influence the course of a disease, see also Prioreschi 1992, 346.

64. Von Staden 1990, 77–84, 99–102.

65. E.g., case 31 of the Egyptian Edwin Smith papyrus; and the Hindu Sushruta Samhita and Caraka Samhita. On the Hindu texts and their English translations, see Prioreschi 1992, 345 with nn. 21–22.

66. The god Thoth is said to have given medical skill to men. On Egyptian medicine, see Majno 1975, 69–140; Nunn 1996; Westendorf 1999. A passage in the Edwin Smith papyrus labels in the following way each case that a healer may encounter: "A disease which I shall treat. A disease with which I shall struggle. A disease which I cannot treat" (translated by von Staden [1989, 14 n. 48]). The last label, "A disease which I cannot treat," coupled with the idea that medicine was, for the Egyptians, already complete, implies that the healer himself, rather than the practice of healing, is limited. Presumably only the gods could treat cases beyond the abilities of the human practitioner.

67. VM 2 = 1.572 L.: Ἰητρικὴ δὲ πάλαι πάντα ὑπάρχει, καὶ ἀρχὴ καὶ ὁδὸς εὑρημένη, καθ᾿ ἣν τὰ εὑρημένα πολλά τε καὶ καλῶς ἔχοντα εὕρηται ἐν πολλῷ χρόνῳ, καὶ τὰ λοιπὰ εὑρεθήσεται, ἤν τις ἱκανός τε ἐὼν καὶ τὰ εὑρημένα εἰδὼς, ἐκ τούτων ὁρμώμενος ζητῇ. Jouanna (1990) has published a new edition of the text with commentary; see also Schiefsky 2005 for extensive commentary. Jouanna (1999, App. 3.5) and Schiefsky (2005, 63–64) date this treatise to the late fifth century BC. Hankinson (1992, 55 n. 2) prefers a date in the fourth century BC on linguistic grounds. The concept of scientific progress is strongly evident in Galen; see Hankinson 1994.

68. In the Gorgias, Socrates illustrates the danger of people posing as doctors: he says that it will often be the smoothest talker, not the best doctor, who persuades the people to vote for him (Grg. 456b–c). Amundsen (1977 and 1996 [esp. 35–37]) discusses the lack of a formal method of legitimating true doctors, although he overplays the negative reputation of doctors in the fifth century. Von Staden (1990) and Prioreschi (1992) discuss the dangers posed to a doctor's reputation by tackling untreatable cases; see also Cohn-Haft 1956, 17–18; Jouanna 1999, 107–111. One factor often mentioned in these discussions is that iatrike was under attack; however, there seems to be no evidence for this as early as the fifth century BC, as argued by Dean-Jones 2003, esp. 103–104. On the reputation of doctors in antiquity, see Amundsen 1977; Demand 1993, who cites fourth-century evidence for their negative reputation in Attic oratory.

69. VM 1 = 1.570 L.: Εἰσὶν δὲ δημιουργοὶ, οἱ μὲν φαῦλοι, οἱ δὲ πολλὸν διαφέροντες· ὅπερ, εἰ μὴ ἦν ἰητρικὴ ὅλως, μηδ᾿ ἐν αὐτῇ ἔσκεπτο μηδ᾿ εὕρητο μηδέν, οὐκ ἂν ἦν, ἀλλὰ πάντες ὁμοίως αὐτῆς ἄπειροί τε καὶ ἀνεπιστήμονες ἦσαν. Most doctors, the author claims, are in fact bad (κακοί). All doctors make mistakes, but bad doctors make grave errors and are easily distinguished from good doctors in severe, violent, and dangerous cases, much as the inadequacies of a poor helmsman are made blatantly evident when a major storm suddenly descends (VM 9 = 1.588–590 L.).

70. Jouanna 1999, 110.

71. Pl. Phaed. 268c: Εἰπεῖν ἂν οἶμαι ὅτι μαίνεται ἄνθρωπος, καὶ ἐκ βιβλίου ποθὲν ἀκούσας ἢ περιτυχὼν φαρμακίοις ἰατρὸς οἴεται γεγονέναι, οὐδὲν ἐπαίων τῆς τέχνης. Also Aristotle (NE 1181b) says that medical treatises are of benefit to those with experience (ἐμπείροις) but useless to those without such knowledge (ἀνεπιστήμοσιν).

72. De arte 9 = 6.16 L.: Δύνανται δὲ οἷσι τά τε τῆς παιδείης μὴ ἐκποδὼν τά τε τῆς φύσιος μὴ ταλαίπωρα.

73. Xen. Mem. 4.2.5.

74. The date is disputed. Erotian attributes it to Hippocrates; Jouanna (1999, App. 3.35) adduces linguistic evidence in support of a date later than the fifth century. Lex 1–2 = 4.638–640 L.: Πρόστιμον γὰρ ἰητρικῆς μούνης ἐν τῇσι πόλεσιν οὐδὲν ὥρισται, πλὴν ἀδοξίης· . . . οὕτω καὶ οἱ ἰητροί, φήμῃ μὲν πολλοί, ἔργῳ δὲ πάγχυ βαιοί. Χρὴ γάρ, ὅστις μέλλει ἰητρικῆς σύνεσιν ἀτρεκέως ἁρμόζεσθαι, τῶνδέ μιν ἐπήβολον γενέσθαι· φύσιος· διδασκαλίης· τόπου εὐφυέος· παιδομαθίης· φιλοπονίης· χρόνου. . . . ἢν μετὰ φρονήσιος δεῖ περιποιήσασθαι, παιδομαθέα γενόμενον ἐν τόπῳ ὁκοῖος εὐφυὴς πρὸς μάθησιν ἔσται.

75. Lex 5 = 4.642 L.: "Holy matters are revealed to holy men. It is not right to reveal them to the uninitiated until they have completed the secret rites of this specialized knowledge." (Τὰ δὲ ἱερὰ ἐόντα πρήγματα ἱεροῖσιν ἀνθρώποισι δείκνυται· βεβήλοισι δὲ οὐ θέμις, πρὶν ἢ τελεσθῶσιν ὀργίοισιν ἐπιστήμης.) Many ancient cults had secret initiatory rites; see Burkert 1987.

76. Pl. Prt. 311b–c: "If, for example, you had thought of going to Hippocrates of Kos, the Asclepiad, and were about to give him your money, and some one had said to you: You are paying money to your namesake Hippocrates, O Hippocrates; tell me, what is he that you give him money? How would you have answered? I should say, he replied, that I gave money to him as a physician." Trans. Benjamin Jowett, in Buchanan 1977, 48. (ὥσπερ ἂν εἰ ἐπενόεις παρὰ τὸν σαυτοῦ ὁμώνυμον ἐλθὼν Ἱπποκράτη τὸν Κῷον, τὸν τῶν Ἀσκληπιαδῶν, ἀργύριον τελεῖν ὑπὲρ σαυτοῦ μισθὸν ἐκείνῳ, εἴ τίς σε ἤρετο· Εἰπέ μοι, μέλλεις τελεῖν, ὦ Ἱππόκρατες, Ἱπποκράτει μισθὸν ὡς τίνι ὄντι;" τί ἂν ἀπεκρίνω;—Εἶπον ἂν, ἔφη, ὅτι ὡς ἰατρῷ.)

77. Nutton 1995c, 19. For bibliography and an overview of the scholarly debate about these schools, see also Langholf 1990.

78. Nutton 1995c; this article is a well-documented and engaging description of medical education and society in the Greek and Roman worlds. Nutton concludes that medical education should be thought of in terms of family units, whether literal or metaphorical, rather than formal institutions.

79. Nutton 1995c, 13–15, lists evidence from Asia Minor and Italy for large numbers of doctors in relatively small towns. He mentions, for example, a third-century BC curse tablet from Metaponto listing the names of no fewer than seventeen Greek doctors (SEG 30.1175). This number is remarkably high given an estimated population of six to seven thousand for this Greek colony in the third century BC.

80. Cf. On the Art. The ease with which anyone could set up shop as a healer (but not as a doctor) is suggested by the following anecdote about Antiphon, the famous fifth-century orator. According to Plutarch, although Antiphon never claimed to be a doctor, he did claim before beginning his career as an orator "to be able to cure distress, just as the treatment of doctors is effective on those who are ill; and setting up a room

near the agora in Corinth, he wrote on the door that he was able to cure those who were troubled. . . . But, believing this *techne* unworthy of him, he turned to rhetoric" (Plut. Mor. 833c–d); see also Jouanna 1999, 77–78. Nutton (1995c, 18 and n. 82) explains that in the Roman period by the time of Pliny one could watch operations taking place on a street corner or in a theater.

Two • Searching for a Cure

1. Morb.Sacr. 1 = 6.358 L.: Προσποιέονται πλέον τι εἰδέναι, καὶ ἀνθρώπους ἐξαπατῶσι προστιθέμενοι αὐτοῖς ἁγνείας τε καὶ καθάρσιας, ὅ τε πολὺς αὐτοῖς τοῦ λόγου ἐς τὸ θεῖον ἀφῆκει καὶ τὸ δαιμόνιον. Καίτοι ἔμοιγε οὐ περὶ εὐσεβείης τοὺς λόγους δοκέουσι ποιεῖσθαι, ὡς οἴονται, ἀλλὰ περὶ ἀσεβείης μᾶλλον, καὶ ὡς οἱ θεοὶ οὐκ εἰσί, τὸ δὲ εὐσεβὲς αὐτῶν καὶ τὸ θεῖον ἀσεβές ἐστι καὶ ἀνόσιον, ὡς ἐγὼ διδάξω.

2. Morb.Sacr. 18 = 6.394 L.: Αὕτη δὲ ἡ νοῦσος ἡ ἱερὴ καλεομένη ἀπὸ τῶν αὐτῶν προφασίων γίνεται ἀφ᾽ ὧν καὶ αἱ λοιπαὶ ἀπὸ τῶν προσιόντων καὶ ἀπιόντων, καὶ ψύχεος καὶ ἡλίου καὶ πνευμάτων μεταβαλλομένων τε καὶ οὐδέποτε ἀτρεμιζόντων. ταῦτα δ᾽ ἐστὶ θεῖα.

3. On the concept of the divine in the Hippocratic corpus, see Thivel 1975 (who, on this very point, also compares Hippocratic medicine to medicine in other ancient cultures); Jouanna 1989; Hankinson 1998b; also van der Eijk 1990 and Jouanna 2003 (focusing on *On the Sacred Disease*), and van der Eijk 1991 (focusing on *Airs, Waters, Places* and *On the Sacred Disease*).

4. Aer. 22 = 2.76–78 L.: Ἐμοὶ δὲ καὶ αὐτῷ δοκεῖ ταῦτα τὰ πάθεα θεῖα εἶναι καὶ τἄλλα πάντα καὶ οὐδὲν ἕτερον ἑτέρου θειότερον οὐδὲ ἀνθρωπινώτερον, ἀλλὰ πάντα ὁμοῖα καὶ πάντα θεῖα. ἕκαστον δὲ αὐτῶν ἔχει φύσιν τὴν ἑωυτοῦ καὶ οὐδὲν ἄνευ φύσιος γίνεται.

5. I owe much of my discussion of this passage to the insights of Dale Martin (2004, 41–45).

6. Morb.Sacr. 1 = 6.362 L.: Οὓς ἐχρῆν τἀναντία τούτων ποιεῖν, θύειν τε καὶ εὔχεσθαι καὶ ἐς τὰ ἱερὰ φέροντας ἱκετεύειν τοὺς θεούς· νῦν δὲ τούτων μὲν ποιέουσιν οὐδέν, καθαίρουσι δέ. Καὶ τὰ μὲν τῶν καθαρμῶν γῆ κρύπτουσι, τὰ δὲ ἐς θάλασσαν ἐμβάλλουσι, τὰ δὲ ἐς τὰ ὄρεα ἀποφέρουσιν, ὅπη μηδεὶς ἄψεται μηδὲ ἐμβήσεται· τὰ δ᾽ ἐχρῆν ἐς τὰ ἱερὰ φέροντας τῷ θεῷ ἀποδοῦναι, εἰ δὴ ὁ θεός ἐστιν αἴτιος.

7. Morb.Sacr. 1 = 6.362 L.: Οὐ μέντοι ἔγωγε ἀξιῶ ὑπὸ θεοῦ ἀνθρώπου σῶμα μιαίνεσθαι, τὸ ἐπικηρότατον ὑπὸ τοῦ ἁγνοτάτου. The most basic meaning of ἐπικηρότατον is "perishable," but in this context it seems to take on the meaning "impure" because of the contrast with ἁγνότατος. The idea that the body is impure or corruptible in contrast to the soul is common in Plato.

8. Modern editions divide *Regimen* into four books, but there was dispute even in antiquity about its division; see Jouanna 1999, 408–409. Jouanna dates Book 4 to the late fifth or fourth century BC; Hankinson (1998b, 16 n. 30) to ca. 400 BC. The author distinguishes between divine and non-divine dreams: divine dreams are from the gods and have their own interpreters, whereas dreams that are not divine result from excesses of or changes to the body during the day, which in turn affect the soul while one sleeps (Vict. IV 87 = 6.640–642 L.). These latter dreams can be interpreted by doctors since they arise from the body. Evidence of the author's piety is reinforced by the very last sentence of the treatise: "Employing

these methods as described will produce a healthy life; and I have discovered regimen, inasmuch as it is possible for a man to do so, with the help of the gods" (Τούτοισι χρώμενος ὡς γέγραπται, ὑγιανεῖ τὸν βίον, καὶ εὕρηταί μοι δίαιτα ὡς δυνατὸν εὑρεῖν ἄνθρωπον ἐόντα ξὺν τοῖσι θεοῖσιν, Vict. IV 93 = 6.662 L.). On the relationship between therapy and the gods posited in this treatise, and the rationality of this view, see also van der Eijk 2004.

9. Vict. IV 89 = 6.652 L.: Περὶ μὲν οὖν τῶν οὐρανίων σημείων οὕτω γινώσκοντα χρὴ προμηθεῖσθαι καὶ ἐκδιαιτῆσαι καὶ τοῖσι θεοῖσιν εὔχεσθαι, ἐπὶ μὲν τοῖσι ἀγαθοῖσι Ἡλίῳ, Διὶ οὐρανίῳ, Διὶ κτησίῳ, Ἀθηνᾷ κτησίῃ, Ἑρμῇ, Ἀπόλλωνι, ἐπὶ δὲ τοῖσι ἐναντίοισι τοῖσι ἀποτροπαίοισι, καὶ Γῆ καὶ ἥρωσιν, ἀποτρόπαια τὰ χαλεπὰ εἶναι πάντα.

10. Vict. IV 90 = 6.656–658 L.: Οὐδὲ μέλαιναν ὁρῆν τὴν γῆν οὐδὲ κατακεκαυμένην ἀγαθόν. . . . εὔχεσθαι δὲ Γῆ καὶ Ἑρμῇ καὶ ἥρωσιν.

11. The author Book I of *Regimen* accepts *mantike* as a *techne* attributed to the mind of the gods (Vict. I 12 = 6.488 L.); see also Hankinson 1998b, 29.

12. Vict. IV 87 = 6.642 L.: Καὶ τὸ μὲν εὔχεσθαι ἀγαθόν· δεῖ δὲ καὶ αὐτὸν συλλαμβάνοντα τοὺς θεοὺς ἐπικαλεῖσθαι.

13. Other passages in the corpus also refer to matters divine, including the prologues to *Prognostic* (fifth century BC) and *Nature of Women* (this prologue is possibly the work of a later editor and based on a passage in *Diseases of Women* 2.3). Thivel (1975, 76) argues that these two references to the divine are traditional formulas (without influence on medicine) that the physicians preserved at the beginning of their discourses. Chapter 6 of *Decorum*, a corrupt passage, seems to attribute much that is positive in medicine to the gods (its date is disputed: late fourth or early third century BC, Thivel 1975; first or second century AD, Jouanna 1999).

14. We find in later sources, like Aelius Aristides in the second century AD, that doctors and Asklepios disagreed as to the proper treatment of certain ailments. One of the most famous examples of the latter is Asklepios telling Aristides in the dead of winter to bathe in a cold stream (*Orat.* 48.20–21). Friends and doctors come to watch, out of concern and curiosity; after Aristides emerges healthy from the river, one doctor admits to having thought Aristides would be lucky to survive the cold plunge with nothing worse than back trouble. But more significant is the fact that Aelius Aristides consulted both doctors and Asklepios, often for the same malady, and never abandoned the one type of healer wholly for the other. On Aristides' consultation of both doctors and Asklepios, as well as other healing gods, see Chapter 3 below.

15. Dean-Jones (1995, 45) argues that since authors of the Hippocratic corpus are vociferous about types of healing with which they disagree, their silence regarding other healers (such as women, in this case) may be interpreted as a sign of their lack of disagreement.

16. The author of *Regimen* 4 seems to be saying that prayer to the gods is to be used not only by those turned away by doctors, but also by those who are under medical treatment. Hankinson (1998b, 11) comments that whatever the degree of personal piety of the authors of the treatises, these suggestions "are clearly invitations to step outside the borders of the practice, not reflections of something integral to it." It is worth noting that all such invitations to step outside the borders of the practice apply to the gods, prayer, sacrifice, and temple-healing; none point specifically to magic, purifiers, etc.

17. Fashioned from materials like clay, wood, marble, and metal, anatomical votives represent the part of the body in need of healing. On Minoan peak sanctuaries, see Peatfield 1990; Nowicki 1994; Jones 1999.

18. As Kearns (1989, 14) observes, almost any god can function as a healer. There is no recent comprehensive study of the healing gods, but see the detailed overview by J.H. Croon, "Heilgötter," in *RAC* 13.1190–1231. Jayne 1925 is still a valuable reference but now incomplete, as is Farnell 1921, which includes some of the healing heroes. Forsén 1996, a study of anatomical votives, provides general information on many Greek healing deities.

19. On anatomical votives in the Greek world, see van Straten 1981, esp. 105–151; Forsén 1996. On the Ephesus votives, many of which were found either in foundations or placed carefully among the blocks of a structure built ca. 700 BC, see Hogarth 1908. On the Artemis votives, which are in the form of hands, see Forsén 1996, 137 with n. 19. On the Hera votives, see Burkert 1992a, 75–79. Gula is also called *azugallatu*, or "the great physician." Burkert ties this Babylonian healing goddess to Asklepios via the presence of dogs in both cults, as well as the similarity of the "*azugallatu*" and "Asklepios." The origin of the name Asklepios has defied explanation, as Burkert explains. On Mesopotamian healing and the cult of Gula and their relation to the cult of Asklepios, see Avalos 1995, 99–231.

20. On healing heroes, see Verbanck-Piérard 2000, in addition to Farnell 1921 and Jayne 1925. On Attic healing heroes, see Kutsch 1913; Kearns 1989, 14–21; Verbanck-Piérard 2000; Gorrini 2001; Gorrini 2005; Vikela 2006; also Chapter 3 below.

21. KA, s.v. "Aristophanes," fr. 22, 28. On Amphiaraos as a healer, see also Chapter 3 below. The tradition of Herakles as an averter of plague may be late; see Keesling 2005, 67–70 with n. 90.

22. Paus. 2.17.8; also Farnell 1896–1909, vol. 4, p. 235–238; Lambrinoudakis 1982; Peppa-Papaioannou 1985; Lambrinoudakis 2002; Riethmüller 2005, vol. 1, 152–157. Asklepios was incorporated into cults of Apollo at many other sites as well, including Corinth and Kos.

23. For a general overview of the history and architecture of Epidauros, see Burford 1969, 41–87; Tomlinson 1983. For further bibliography, see Riethmüller 2005, vol. 1, 148–174, 279–324; Melfi 2007, 17–209. On the recent excavations, see Lambrinoudakis 2002, who mentions (220) the presence of prehistoric, geometric, and early Archaic pottery sherds near an early well but cautions that these may have been brought from the Maleatas sanctuary to consecrate the new site. The inscription to Apollo is at *IG* IV² 1 142, that to Asklepios at *IG* IV² 1 136. Jeffrey 1990, 179–181 dates both to ca. 500 BC based on the alphabet and letter forms.

24. See Edelstein and Edelstein 1945, vol. 2, 208–213, for discussion of games in honor of Asklepios. Pindar's death ca. 438 BC provides a *terminus ante quem* for his odes. Moreover, in *Nemean* 5, Pindar says that the grandfather of the boy to whom the ode is addressed won a victory in the *pankration* at Epidauros, indicating that this contest took place by the early fifth century (if not earlier), about two generations before the composition of the ode; see Edelstein and Edelstein 1945, vol. 2, 208.

25. Ancient commentators on Pindar mention no one other than Asklepios as honorand of these games: Schol. ad *Nem.* 5.95–96, *Nem.* 3.84. Not all scholars agree, however,

that these games had ties to the cult of Asklepios; for discussion, see Edelstein and Edelstein 1945, vol. 2, 208–209.

26. The dramatic date of this dialogue is uncertain, but it must be before the time of Socrates' death, in 399 BC.

27. Strabo 14.1.39 (C 647), Hyg. *Fab.* 14.21, and Euseb. *Praep.Ev.* 3.14.6 all say that Asklepios is from Trikka; *Il.* 2.729–733 and 4.198–202 identify Machaon and Podaleirios as coming from Trikka; cf. Eustath. *Il.* 2.729, 4.202. Solimano 1976 discusses the various geographical traditions for the myth of Asklepios.

28. The Trikkan coin, ca. 400-350 BC, depicts the nymph Trikka on the obverse and on the reverse a male who may be Asklepios, seated, feeding a serpent, with a staff against his shoulder and a bird in his right hand. See *LIMC*, s.v. "Asklepios," no. 52 with plate; and *BMC* vol. 6, *Thessaly to Aetolia*, p. 52, no. 17 = *LIMC*, s.v. "Asklepios," no. 40 with plate, for another, very similar coin of the same period also from Trikka. The Larissan coin, ca. 450–400 BC, depicts a horse on the obverse and on the reverse a male who may be Asklepios, feeding a serpent (*BMC* vol. 6, *Thessaly to Aetolia*, p. 28, no. 44;). If Percy Gardner's date in *BMC* is correct for this coin, there may have been a cult of Asklepios at Larissa by the fifth century. It is often difficult on coins to differentiate Asklepios from certain other male deities, especially Apollo; see Penn 1994, 19–20, 46. For this reason, none of the coins cited in this note can be said with certainty to depict Asklepios. Excavators have identified a site at Trikka as an Asklepieion on tentative material evidence. On Asklepieia in Thessaly, including Trikka, see Melfi 2003, 418–437; Riethmüller 2005, vol. 1, 91–106, vol. 2, 289–315.

29. Anaxilas lived 494–476 BC. See Thucy. 6.4.6; and the article by David Asheri in *CAH²*, vol. 4, ch. 16.

30. This sanctuary has not yet been recovered. For sources and bibliography, see Riethmüller 2005, vol. 2, 72–73 no. 25.

31. SEG 25.226; see also Chapter 4 below. According to the inscription, Asklepios came to Athens via Zea harbor, which suggests to some that a sanctuary of Asklepios was in place at Piraeus by then (e.g., Burford 1969, 25–26 and 51) or that a sanctuary was established there in 420 during the cult's transfer to Athens (e.g., Garland 2001, 115). Parker (1996, 181–182) cautions against these interpretations since there is no certain evidence for the Piraeus cult before the fourth century BC. Evidence for the cult is discussed by Semeria 1986, 943; Garland 2001, esp. 208 n. 115, and Appendix III, s.v. "Asklepios"; von Eickstedt 2001; Riethmüller 2005, vol. 2, 25–35 no. 10.

32. On the archaeology and history of the sanctuary of Asklepios at Corinth, see Roebuck 1951; Lang 1977 (the latter is a brief overview). For recent discussion, sources, and bibliography, see Riethmüller 2005, vol. 1, 123–130; Melfi 2007, 289–312.

33. Roebuck 1951, 14–15, and cat. no. 1.

34. Roebuck 1951, 111–151: These anatomical votives were probably dedicated to Asklepios rather than Apollo since Asklepios' name appears on pottery associated with them (see also Roebuck 152–153), but we cannot be certain.

35. The dating of individual Asklepieia based on little more than inference from a work of art is highly speculative inasmuch as it assumes that (1) the sculptors named by Pausanias and Strabo are the same as those known to us as fifth–century artists, and (2)

these statues were originally designed for these sanctuaries. Ancient sources indicate that sculptors named Kalamis and Kolotes lived in later centuries; see Pollitt 1990. And Pausanias himself records the transfer of bronze and wood statues from sanctuary to sanctuary (Paus. 8.30.3; 8.31.5). The statue at Sikyon was gold and ivory, that at Kyllene ivory. Pausanias does not mention the material of the Mantinean statue, but even if it were marble, its weight would not have prevented its transfer. There is, moreover, a related problem of matching what Pausanias describes as a statue by a certain sculptor with what is known otherwise to be typical of that artist's style; see the comments of Holtzmann in LIMC, s.v. "Asklepios," esp. no. 890. For ancient sources and bibliography pertaining to these sites, see Riethmüller 2005, vol. 2, 208–213 no. 92 (Mantinea); vol. 1, 130–133, vol. 2, 63–68 no. 23 (Sikyon); vol. 2, 170–171 no. 75 (Kyllene).

36. PECS, s.v. "Epidauros." The problem with estimates like this is determining exactly which cults of Asklepios are being included in the estimate, and upon what evidence that dating is made. Dating, as noted above, is often based on the name of an artist who sculpted a statue mentioned by Pausanias or Strabo. Ancient sources, bibliography, and discussion of evidence for Asklepieia in Greece is compiled by Semeria 1986; Melfi 2003 and 2007; Riethmüller 2005 (who also catalogues the information for Asklepieia outside Greece). On Asklepieia in the Peloponnese, see also Stavropoulos 1996; Gorrini 2003.

37. At least two cities in antiquity are said to have consulted Delphi regarding the importation of Asklepios: Halieis (IG IV² 1 122.69–82 = LiDonnici 1995 [B 33]) and Rome (Ov. Met. 15.626–643). There were also links between Delphi and Hippocrates of Kos. Pausanias reports that a statue at Delphi of a man whose body was decaying from illness was, according to the Delphians, dedicated by Hippocrates (Paus. 10.2.6). In pseudo-Hippocrates, Hippocrates traveled to Delphi during the great plague and asked Apollo to save the Greeks. As a result, the Asklepiads were given the right of promanteia, priority in consulting the oracle (Hipp. Ep. 27.7).

38. For ancient sources and bibliography pertaining to these Asklepieia, see Riethmüller 2005. On the spread of Asklepios' cult in the Roman world, see Degrassi 1986; Musial 1992; Tiussi 1999; Renberg 2006/2007. On Greco-Roman Asklepieia, see also Graf 1992.

39. Athens: Travlos 1971, s.v. "Asklepieion"; Lefantzis and Jensen, forthcoming. For Corinth: Roebuck 1951, esp. 23–26, for description and dates of the early Hellenistic buildings; Melfi 2007, 23–63.

40. See LiDonnici 1995, 10–14, for a brief summary of the fourth-century building program. For a more detailed description and bibliography, including analysis of the fourth-century building accounts, see Burford 1969; also Riethmüller 2005, vol. 1, 279–324, with references.

41. IG IV² 1 94 and 1.95. On theorodokoi in the Peloponnese and for discussion of these decrees, see Perlman 2000, esp. 67–97 on Epidauros.

42. See Roebuck 1951, 113–138; on the Asklepios inscriptions, see also Roebuck 1951, nos. 61 and 65–67.

43. On the votive reliefs, see LIMC, s.v. "Asklepios"; also Holländer 1912; Hausmann 1948; Comella 2002, 46–56 (fifth-century reliefs), 102–112 (fourth-century reliefs). The

reliefs are being restudied by Jesper Jensen for his Ph.D. dissertation, "The Votive Reliefs from the Athenian Asklepieion on the South Slope of the Akropolis" (University of Aarhus, Denmark). The inventory lists, which date from the fourth to second centuries BC, were studied by Aleshire (1989).

44. LiDonnici 1995, 50–75, analyzes probable sources for the narratives.

45. It is uncertain which sanctuary of Asklepios is described by Aristophanes. The scholiast to the *Ploutos* says that it is the sanctuary on the Acropolis (ἐν ἄστει) in Athens (*ad loc.* 621). Scholars have doubted this assertion, however, mainly because the sanctuary in the *Ploutos* is described as being near the sea (Pl. 656–658). For this reason, many believe that the Asklepieion in the *Ploutos* is the sanctuary at Zea in Piraeus. Asklepios appears also in tragedy and epinician in the late sixth century and fifth century, but it is difficult to read these accounts as certain references to the cult. According to the Suda, Aristarchos of Tegea wrote a tragedy entitled *Asklepios* in thanks for being cured by the god (Snell 1971 [F 14.1]), but this may reflect a later tradition. One further genre deserves mention here: paeans honoring the god were performed at sanctuaries of Asklepios probably by the late fifth century when musical contests were held at Epidauros. Ancient tradition ascribes to Sophocles a paean in honor of Asklepios (Lucian *Demosthenes Encomium* 27; Philostr. VA 3.17; also SEG 28.225 = IG II² 4510). On this paean, see also Chapter 4 below.

46. P.Didot = P.Louvre 7172. For text, translation, and discussion of this papyrus fragment, see G.W. Arnott 2000, 473–479.

47. The Greek original is unknown. For Plautus' innovations on the presumed original, see Moore 1998, 126–139.

48. KA, "Antiphanes," fr. 47, "Philetaerus," fr. 1–2. Menander was Athenian and many of his plays were performed in Athens, but it is hard to believe that his one hundred–plus plays could all have been performed at Athenian festivals; see Sandbach 1977, 70–73; G.W. Arnott 1979, vol. 1, xiv–xvi.

49. Early evidence from the sanctuary at Epidauros provides no unambiguous indication of healing. The stoas of a structure known as Building E prompted Robert (1933, 391) to conclude that incubation was part of early cult activity there, but Tomlinson (1983, 74–75) cautions against this interpretation, citing two factors in particular: the ash debris from the altar in the courtyard of Building E does not necessarily imply that Building E itself was a hallowed building, and Building E does not give any indication of what its own ritual function may have been. A stoa is a very practical structure providing protection from sun and rain, and, as Tomlinson (1992) urges in his interpretation of the sanctuary of Hera at Perachora, greater consideration must be given to the practical needs of the worshippers alongside their often-exaggerated ritual needs. Lambrinoudakis (2002, 219) suggests that a sixth-century stoa under the later stoa was used for incubation, but he bases this assumption on proximity to a nearby well and the presumed function of the later stoa.

50. LiDonnici (1995, 76–82) convincingly argues that some of the healing experiences inscribed on Stele A in the mid-fourth century BC reflect votives and visits to the sanctuary in the fifth century. Her arguments are based on linguistic characteristics and references within the inscriptions to earlier inscriptions. I am not convinced, however,

that the healing events and votives date to the *beginning* of the fifth century BC, as she claims. For other *iamata* from Epidauros, as well as *iamata* from Athens, Lebena, Pergamon, and Rome, see Girone 1998.

51. Broken vessel: IG IV² 1 121.79–89 = LiDonnici 1995 (A10); missing treasure: IG IV² 1 123.8–21 = LiDonnici 1995 (C3); lost oil bottle: IG IV² 1 123.129–134 = LiDonnici 1995 (C22); lost child: IG IV² 1 122.19–26 = LiDonnici 1995 (B4). Punishment: IG IV² 1 121.33–41 = LiDonnici 1995 (A4), IG IV² 1 122.7–9 = LiDonnici 1995 (B2), and IG IV² 1 122.95–101 = LiDonnici 1995 (B16).

52. IG IV² 1 121.2 = LiDonnici 1995, stele A: [ἰά]ματα τοῦ Ἀπόλλωνος καὶ τοῦ Ἀσκλαπιοῦ.

53. The tenth narrative, which refers to Asklepios, is IG IV² 1 121.79–89 = LiDonnici 1995 (A10). On the chronology and grouping of the narratives, see LiDonnici 1995, 20–82.

54. See also LiDonnici 1995, 46 n. 28. The same may have been true at Corinth by the late fifth century. As noted above, however, whether the Corinthian votives were dedicated to Apollo or Asklepios is uncertain.

55. On pilgrims to Asklepios at Epidauros, see Dillon 1994, 243; and Dillon 1997, 73–80.

56. Aleshire 1989, 71. Also Aleshire 1992.

Three • Asklepios and His Colleagues

1. At *Od.* 4.232, Helen's comment that all physicians in Egypt are descendants of Paieon suggests that this tradition is novel to her immediate audience and probably also to Homer's larger audience.

2. The brief, five-line *Homeric Hymn to Asklepios* also identifies Asklepios as the son of Apollo. The hymn, however, provides too little in the way of content or style to make it datable; see Janko 1982, 1.

3. Asklepios' training is attested in, e.g., Pind. *Nem.* 3.54–56, *Pyth.* 3.1–7; Xen. *Cyn.* 1.1–6; Philostr. *Her.* 9; Heraclit. *All.* 15.

4. On sources for Asklepios' punishment and death, see Edelstein and Edelstein 1945, vol. 1, T. 105–115; Gantz 1993, 91–92. Apollo's servitude to Admetus is most famously portrayed in Euripides' *Alkestis*. When and how Asklepios attained immortality after dying is not explained in ancient accounts until late antiquity; see Edelstein and Edelstein 1945, vol. 2, 67–76. The fragmentary nature of Hesiod's account leaves uncertain whether he envisioned such a destiny for Asklepios. It is tempting to associate his apotheosis with a remark in *On Ancient Medicine* that the first researchers of medicine believed their *techne* worthy of being ascribed to a god (VM 14 = 1.600–602 L.). Perhaps this desire to ascribe developments in medicine to a famous and even immortal personage prompted the apotheosis sometime between Homer and Pindar.

5. Exactly whom Asklepios raised from the dead was a matter debated already in the fifth century BC; candidates include Hippolytus, Glaukos, Tyndareos, Hymenaeus, Capaneus, Lykourgos, "the dead in Delphi," the Phinidae, Orion, and the daughters of Proteus.

6. The Greek text is that of C.M. Bowra (Oxford Classical Texts).

7. See Graf 1997, 28–29 with n. 29; Furley 1993, 80–104. The noun *epaoidos* is used twice elsewhere in Pindar: *Nem.* 8.49 and *Pyth.* 4.217; in the latter it appears in the context of Medea's sorcery. On the use of incantations and other utterances to establish a healer's authority, see Gordon 1995. Kotansky (1991, 108–110) and Scarborough (1991, 143) assume that παράπτων φάρμακα at *Pyth.* 3.52–53 describes Asklepios affixing amulets. This is certainly possible, although the same phrase may also connote the application of poultices to the skin. There is ambiguity about the use of incantations by doctors in Sophocles' *Ajax*: a wise doctor does not sing incantations over a pain that requires surgery (οὐ πρὸς ἰατροῦ σοφοῦ / θρηνεῖν ἐπῳδὰς πρὸς τομῶντι πήματι, *Aj.* 581–582; text of H. Lloyd-Jones and N.G. Wilson, Oxford Classical Texts). This implies either that doctors never used *epaoidoi*, or that there is a right and wrong time for their use, even by the wise doctor. A reading in favor of the former finds support in the boar-wound episode at *Od.* 19.455–462 where Odysseus' wound is treated with incantations but the healers are not called doctors.

8. See the discussions in Edelstein and Edelstein 1945, vol. 2, 112; Lloyd 1979, 37–49.

9. Drugs for the eyes: IG IV² 1 121.33–41 = LiDonnici 1995 (A4), IG IV² 1 121.72–78 = LiDonnici 1995 (A9); removal and attachment of body parts: IG IV² 1 122.1–6 = LiDonnici 1995 (B1), IG IV² 1 122.10–19 = LiDonnici 1995 (B3); belly surgery: IG IV² 1 122.10–19 = LiDonnici 1995 (B3), IG IV² 1 122.26–35 = LiDonnici 1995 (B5); removal of material from the belly: IG IV² 1 122.26–35 = LiDonnici 1995 (B5); draining of fluids: IG IV² 1 122.1–6 = LiDonnici 1995 (B1). On the dating of these healing experiences, see LiDonnici 1995, 76–82.

10. Incubation by proxy, as in this instance, is unusual in Asklepios' cult. IG IV² 1 122.1–6 = LiDonnici 1995 (B1): Ἀράτα [Λά]καινα ὕδρωπ[α. ὑπ]ὲρ ταύτας ἁ μάτηρ ἐνεκάθ-ευδεν ἐλ Λακεδαίμονι ἔσσα[ς] καὶ ἐνύπνιον [ὁ]ρῆι· ἐδόκει τᾶς θυγατρός οὐ τὸν θεὸν ἀποταμόντα τὰν κ[ε]φαλὰν τὸ σῶμα κραμάσαι κάτω τὸν τράχαλον ἔχον· ὡς δ' ἐξερρύα συχνὸν ὑγρ[ό]ν, καταλύσαντα τὸ σῶμα τὰν κεφαλὰν πάλιν ἐπιθέμεν ἐπὶ τὸν αὐχένα· ἰδο[ῦ]σα δὲ τὸ ἐνύπνιον τοῦτο ἀγχωρήσασα εἰς Λακεδαίμονα καταλαμβάνε[ι τ]ὰν θυγατέρα ὑγιαίνουσαν καὶ τὸ αὐτὸ ἐνύπνιον ὡρακυῖαν.

11. On parallels between Hippocratic theory and this particular cure, see also Tinker 1983, 84. Suspension by the feet is a medical procedure: in *Mul.* 3.248 = 8.462 L. it is used to treat a prolapse of the womb; see also King 1998, 160.

12. Dogs: IG IV² 1 121.113–119 = LiDonnici 1995 (A17); IG IV² 1 121.125–126 = LiDonnici 1995 (A20); IG IV² 1 122.35–38 = LiDonnici 1995 (B6). Snakes: IG IV² 1 122.102–110 = LiDonnici 1995 (B17); IG IV² 1 122.117–119 = LiDonnici 1995 (B19); IG IV² 1 122.128–131 = LiDonnici 1995 (B22); IG IV² 1 123.1–3 = LiDonnici 1995 (C1); IG IV² 1 123.104–108 = LiDonnici 1995 (C2); IG IV² 1 123.89–94 = LiDonnici 1995 (C15). Horses: IG IV² 1 122.110–116 = LiDonnici 1995 (B18). Geese: IG IV² 1 122.132–133 = LiDonnici 1995 (B23).

13. IG IV² 1 121.113–119 = LiDonnici 1995 (A17): ἀνὴρ δάκτυλον ἰάθη ὑπὸ ὄφιος, οὗτος τὸν τοῦ ποδὸς δάκτυλον ὑπὸ του ἀγρίου ἕλκεος δεινῶς διακείμενος μεθάμερα ὑπὸ τῶν θεραπόντων ἐξενειχθεὶς ἐπὶ ἐδράματός τινος καθῖζε· ὕπνου δέ νιν λαβόντος ἐν τούτωι δράκων ἐκ τοῦ ἀβάτου ἐξελθὼν τὸν δάκτυλον ἰάσατο τᾶι γλώσσαι καὶ τοῦτο ποιήσας εἰς τὸ ἄβατον ἀνεχώρησε πάλιν. ἐξεγερθεὶς δὲ ὡς ἦς ὑγιής, ἔφα ὄψιν ἰδεῖν, δοκεῖν νεανίσκον εὐπρεπῆ τὰμ μορφὰν ἐπὶ τὸν δάκτυλον ἐπιπῆν φάρμακον.

14. If Herzog's reading of IG IV² 1 123.4–8 = LiDonnici 1995 (C2) is correct, another Epidaurian *iama* tells that a tumor (φῦμα) is healed when a snake "opens" it, presumably by biting it (Herzog reads δάγματι ἀνοίγει; Hiller reads ταὶ ἔχιες ἔλειξαν). "Opening" the tumor would cause it to drain, which again sounds much like humoral rebalance. National Archaeological Museum, Athens, inv. no. 3369.

15. Ael. NA 9.33. This account bears a strong resemblance to the cure of Aristagora of Troezen recorded in the Epidaurian *iamata* (IG IV² 1 122.10–19 = LiDonnici 1995 [B3]).

16. For more about illustrations of medical instruments on coins, pottery, and in sculpture, see Berger 1970. For coins, see also Hart 2000.

17. BMC vol. 10, *Peloponnesus*, p. 157, no. 12; also Berger 1970, fig. 83a and 83b.

18. ICr I 17.8–20. On the Cretan *iamata*, see also Weinreich 1909, 111–136; Tinker 1983, 84–85; LiDonnici 1995, 46–49; and Krug 1985, 157–159. Inscriptions from Rome (IGUR 148, second century AD) indicate similar procedures, as well as detailed information about diet and exercise.

19. ICr I 17.9.

20. On Aelius Aristides' close relationship with both doctors and Asklepios, and his knowledge of medicine, see Horstmanshoff 2004. See also n. 54 below.

21. IG IV² 1 122.60–63 = LiDonnici 1995 (B11). It is remarkable that in the *iamata* from Epidauros five of the six women seeking help for matters related to pregnancy are treated in a supernatural way, such as by touch or sleeping with a snake. The only exception is a woman suffering from a false pregnancy, whose stomach is cut open to remove basins full of unspecified creatures; IG IV² 1 122.26–35 = LiDonnici 1995 (B5). On healing by touch in Asklepios' cult, see also Tinker 1983, 54–56.

22. IG IV² 1 121.41–48 = LiDonnici 1995 (A5).

23. Burkert (1985, 214) emphasizes the "complex personalities" of the other gods as compared to the "one single [healing] function" of Asklepios.

24. Weinreich 1909, 41; Jayne 1925, 229. "Hyperdexios" is used for other gods as well, including Zeus and Athena; see L. Robert 1955, 62–66 on its range of potential meanings.

25. On Apollo as *iatros* in Asia Minor and on the Black Sea, see Ehrhardt 1989; Burkert 1994.

26. It is uncertain whether in *Birds* Apollo is meant to treat humans or their sheep and oxen, whose eyes the birds threaten to peck out. Dunbar (1995, *ad loc.*) reads the latter. As early as Aeschylus, Apollo is called an *iatromantis* (*Eum.* 62).

27. Calder 1971.

28. According to Gantz (1993, 96) the assimilation is suggested by Sappho (LP fr. 44) and is certain by Sophocles (OT 145). Homer is emphatic that Paieon healed gods, not men: both times he heals, his patients, Hades and Ares, are further described as being "not by nature mortal" (οὐ μὲν γάρ τι καταθνητός γ' τέτυκτο, Il. 5.402; also Il. 5.901). A Linear B tablet from Knossos mentions Paieon; see Burkert 1985, 43.

29. Stafford (2005, 124) rightly remarks that the particular cures these authors ascribe to Athena (Pliny says Athena prescribed a specific plant called perdicium or parthenium) owe much to healing procedures attested for Asklepios in the second century BC and later.

30. On Attic healing heroes, see Kutsch 1913; Purday 1987; Kearns 1989, 14–21; Verbanck-Piérard 2000; Gorrini 2001; Gorrini 2005; Vikela 2006.

31. On the cult of Amphiaraos, see Petrakos 1968; Schachter 1981–, vol. 1, p. 19–26; Kearns 1989, 14–21 and app. 1, s.v. "Ἀμφιάραος"; Forsén 1996, 146–147; Petrakos 1997; Gorrini 2001, 302–304.

32. See van Straten 1981, 124–125, for a description and analysis of the stele, as well as a brief list of some of the other votives in the same sanctuary.

33. Hdt. 1.46, 1.49, 1.52, 1.92, 8.134. The original location of this cult is contested; see Hubbard 1992, 103–107, on the debate.

34. On the prevalence of the healing as opposed to the mantic function of the cult, see Schachter 1981–, vol. 1, p. 23 n. 7. The places to which Amphiaraos' cult spread include Athens, Rhamnous, and Piraeus; see Kearns 1989, app. 1, s.v. "Ἀμφιάραος" for bibliography. Pouilloux (1954, 143 n. 30) argues that Amphiaraos took over the sanctuary of another healing god at Rhamnous. Votives and inscriptions indicate great cult activity: for inscriptions, see Schwenk 1985, no. 17, 28, 40, 41, 50; and Mikalson 1998, 33; for votives, see Petrakos 1968. On the longevity and overall popularity of the cult in antiquity, see Schachter 1981–, vol. 1, p. 24–25 with nn. 2 and 3. On the establishment of the cult as occurring after the arrival of Asklepios, and on early procedures for incubation, see Petropoulou 1981.

35. See Purday 1987, 179–184; Kearns 1989, 14–21 and app. 1, s.v. "Ἥρως ἰατρός"; Forsén 1996, 146; Gorrini 2001, 304–306.

36. Travlos 1971, s.v. "Amyneion," with bibliography; Purday 1987, 69–102; Kearns 1989, 14–21 and app. 1, s.v. "Ἄμυνος"; Forsén 1996, 54–56, 146; Gorrini 2001, 304–305.

37. IG II² 1252, 1253, 4365, 4385, 4422, 4424, 4435.

38. The longevity of Amphiaraos' cult is attested by IG II² 839–840. On the association of Heros Iatros with Amphiaraos' son, see Kearns 1989, s.v. "Ἀμφίλοχος," citing Kutsch 1913, no. 4.

39. Evidence for Athena Hygieia on the Acropolis is tenuous until construction of her statue and altar, which Keesling (2005, following Michaelis 1876) convincingly places after 432 BC. See also the discussion in Stafford 2005.

40. On the walking staff as a component of Asklepios' iconography, see Holtzmann's article in *LIMC*, s.v. "Asklepios," with bibliography. Ancient sources debate the meaning of this staff, but none link it to Asklepios' role as physician; see Edelstein and Edelstein 1945, vol. 2, 227–229. As Ludwig Edelstein points out, however, the connection between the itinerant Asklepios and a walking staff is highly appropriate, given his mythology.

41. The authorship and date of the oath are disputed. Erotian attributed it to Hippocrates, and Galen wrote a commentary on it. It must predate the first century AD, when the first reference to it appears in Scribonius Largus *Comp.* 5. For text and commentary, including discussion of the date, see Edelstein 1943, and Lichtenthaeler 1984.

42. Tzetzes *Chiliades* 12.637–639 explains the distinction. For discussion of Asklepiadae, see W.D. Smith 1990, 9–17; Jouanna 1989, 17–22; Jouanna 1999, 10–12 (with nn. 16 and 17), 33–35. The term "Asklepiadae" first appears in Theognis (432), but the passage may be an interpolation. It also occurs in Euripides (*Alc.* 969); Plato (*Prt.* 311b6;

Phdr. 270c; *Rep.* 3.406a); two inscriptions of the fifth century BC (Delphi Museum, inv. no. 3522; Greek Anthology 7.508); and an inscription from the fourth century BC (Delphi Museum, inv. no. 6687A and B, and no. 8131). See Edelstein and Edelstein 1945, vol. 1, T. 217–231 for other occurrences.

43. On the compilation and publication of the *iamata*, see LiDonnici 1995, 50–75. Gorrini 2005 examines the impact of Hippocratic medicine on Attic healing cults, including that of Asklepios.

44. Athens: IG II² 1533.34, 86–87, 116 (329/8 BC); IG II² 1534A.84a (274/3 BC); IG II² 1534B.155, 161 (244/3 BC). Piraeus: IG II² 47.8–9, 11, 16–19 (ca. 360 BC). Two doctors are mentioned as dedicants on lists of the fourth and third centuries BC; see Aleshire 1989, esp. 44, 65, 71. Medical instruments were also dedicated to Asklepios on the island of Delos: ID 1414.9 (second century BC); ID 1416A II.9-10 (second century BC). On the Delos inventories, see Hamilton 2000, esp. 183–186, 190–191. On medical instruments at Asklepieia, see also Wickkiser 2006.

45. Kos: Herzog 1931, 148 with n. 15; Zervos 1932; Sherwin-White 1978, 275 with n. 103. Aleshire 1989, 156, discusses the statue of Polykritos.

46. On the inscription, see also Samama 2003, no. 011. Nutton 1995c, 4, discusses the importance of this ritual to the professionalism of doctors: it functioned as an assertion of their collegiality and of their distinction from other types of healers.

47. Mosaic: Archaeological Museum, Kos. It is discussed by Sherwin-White 1978, 338; Jouanna 1999, 5. Koan coin: BMC vol. 18, *Caria and Islands*, p. 216, no. 216 (dated to the Imperial period); also Berger 1970, fig. 102. On Hippocrates' divine status, see Sherwin-White 1978, 355–356; Temkin 1991, 71–75; Jouanna 1999, 37–38; Zeller 2003. For a text, translation, and discussion of the *Pseudepigraphia*, see W.D. Smith 1990; Pinault 1992.

48. The sources for this evidence are noted by Sherwin-White (1978, 283–285), who describes in detail Xenophon's attachment to Asklepios. For epigraphic evidence concerning Stertinius Xenophon, see also Samama 2003, nos. 142–147. According to Barclay Head (BMC vol. 18, *Caria and Islands*, pp. 215–216, no. 215) the same staff-and-serpent die used for the reverse of Xenophon's coins was also used for those depicting Hippocrates.

49. On the tombs and the medical instruments found therein, see Sherwin-White 1978, 281, items 5–6 with n. 142.

50. Oehler 1909, 16, lists some of the doctors who served as priests. Athens: IG II² 3798.3–5 (date: AD 98/9–103/4); also Aleshire 1989, 59. Aleshire (1989, 74 and 87–88) discusses the office and duties of *zakoroi* and believes that the office may have had something to do with medical treatment for suppliants. Nysa: Sherwin-White 1978, 353 n. 530. Smyrna: IG XIV 967b (ca. AD 200); the desire for the statue to be highly visible is expressed by the clause νηῷ δ᾽ ἐν τῷδε ζωάγρια θῆκεν ὁρᾶσθαι. For further examples, see Nutton 2004, 281.

51. Galen on being a descendant of Asklepios: *San.Tu.* (Kühn 6.41), *Lib. Prop.* (Kühn 19.8–48); healed by Asklepios: *Lib. Prop.* (Kühn 19.8–48), cf. also *Cur.Rat.Ven.Sect.* (Kühn 11.314–315); advice from Asklepios: *Praen.* (Kühn 14.649–651). On the second century AD as a renaissance of Asklepios' cult and on Galen's relationship with Asklepios, see Bowersock 1969, 59–75. On Galen's life, see Nutton 1973, and 2004, 216–229.

52. Galen, MM (Kühn 10.609); Hipp.Hum. (Kühn 16.223); Ord.Lib.Prop. (Kühn 19.59).

53. Bowersock (1969, 74) suggests that Galen's connections to Pergamon and consequently also with Asklepios may have fueled Galen's own prestige. On his position in the cult, see Galen, Lib.Prop. (Kühn 19.19); also Nutton 1973, 162 with n. 4.

54. Aristides even imagined that one of the temple staff from the Asklepieion in Pergamon came to him in a dream in the guise of a physician (Or. 419.25). On Aristides' polytheism, see Behr 1968, 25–27. On his frequent consultation of physicians in conjunction with the commands of Asklepios, see Behr 1968, 44; Tinker 1983, 118–120; Temkin 1991, 184–187. On his religious belief generally, see Kudlien 1981. Pearcy (1992, 609) argues convincingly that doctors in the Sacred Tales serve as foils for Asklepios, but this does not alter the fact that doctors pervade the Sacred Tales, that Aristides consults them alongside Asklepios in his quest for health, and that they are not always in conflict with Asklepios' recommendations, as Behr (1968, 44) points out.

55. King (1999, 283–284) recommends rethinking the traditional model of Asklepios' cult as only an alternative to medicine. She suggests, for example, that doctors might have been an alternative to Asklepios when the latter proved ineffective, but we simply lack the evidence (like healing inscriptions for doctors) to demonstrate this.

56. Medical competitions: I. Eph. 1161–1169, 4101b; see also Edelstein and Edelstein 1945, vol. 2, 212; Nutton 1995c, 7 with n. 23. One such medical kit of the first century AD was made of bronze with silver and niello inlay (Staatliche Museen, Berlin, inv. no. Fr 1222). The ring depicting Asklepios and a doctor: British Museum, inv. no. 1912.3-11.1; another ring depicting Asklepios and Hygieia is illustrated in Simon 1990, fig. 12.

57. IG IV² 1 122.63–68 = LiDonnici 1995 (B12): Ἀ[ντικ]ράτης Κνίδιος ὀφθαλμούς. οὗτος ἔν τινι μάχαι ὑπὸ δό[ρα]τος πλα[γεὶ]ς δι᾽ ἀμφοτέρων τῶν ὀφθαλμῶν τυφλὸς ἐγένετο καὶ τὰν λόγχαν [ἐνε]οῦσαν ἐν τῶι προσώπωι περιέφερε· ἐγκαθεύδων [δ]ὲ ὄψιν εἶδε· ἐδ[όκε]ι οὐ τὸν θεὸν ἐξελκύσαντα τὸ βέλος εἰς τὰ β[λέ]φαρα τὰς καλουμ[έν]ας κόρας πάλιν ἐναρμόξαι· ἀμέρας δὲ γενομένας ὑγιὴς ἐξῆλθ[ε]. On "girls" [κόρας] as referring to pupils, see LiDonnici 109 n. 30.

58. On Asklepios' treatment of chronic rather than fatal conditions, see also Wickkiser 2006. On phthisis, see Hankinson 1995, 55–58, esp. n. 41. Gerald Hart, a medical doctor who has studied Asklepios' cures, argues that many of these cases might have been psychosomatic or responsive to conservative therapy and spontaneous recovery (Hart 2000, 88).

59. For a list in chronological order of the iamata of Epidauros, see LiDonnici 1995, 79.

60. Epidauros: IG IV² I 255.125–127 (second–third century AD); Lebena: ICr I.17.9, 11, 17–19 (second century BC–third century AD); Athens: IG II² 4514 (second century AD); Rome: IGUR I 105, 148; SEG 43.661 (second–third century AD).

61. Kleo: IG IV² 1 121.3–9 = LiDonnici 1995 (A1); Ithmonika: IG IV² 1 121.10–22 = LiDonnici 1995 (A2); Euhippos: IG IV² 1 121.95–97 = LiDonnici 1995 (A12); Gorgias: IG IV² 1 122.55–60 = LiDonnici 1995 (B10).

62. Only two individuals, Galen and Aelius Aristides, claim that Asklepios saved them from death (Gal. Lib.Prop. 18–19; Arist. Or. 50.39–45). Galen states that Asklepios had cured him of a deadly abscess (θανατικὴν διάθεσιν ἀποστήματος). But the context of this statement suggests that it served a diplomatic way out of an unwelcome situation: Galen

tells Marcus Aurelius that he cannot accompany him to the German front because Asklepios, who had once saved him from death, has advised against it. That Galen owes Asklepios his life for curing him of a fatal ailment makes the god's advice on any matter impossible for Galen to ignore. The second individual, Aelius Aristides, thanks Asklepios for saving him from a plague that almost killed him (διηγγέλθη ὡς οἰχησομένου αὐτίκα); but Athena plays a more active role than Asklepios in the narrative of his cure, and her mere presence here (she appears little otherwise in the *Sacred Tales*) suggests that Asklepios alone could not successfully treat this ailment. Asklepios is also credited with ending a plague (typically a fatal condition) that struck Rome in 295 BC, but the earliest sources for this event date from several centuries after the plague, and it is possible that the sources conflate an actual plague with other threats to the body politic; see Wickkiser 2003, chs. 7–9.

63. *Anth.Pal.* 6.330 (plausibly also identified with a very fragmentary inscription at Epidauros, *IG* IV² 1 255): "Having despaired of the skill of mortals, but with every hope in the divine, having left Athens with its many offspring, I came to your grove, Asklepios, and in three months was healed of an ulcer that I had on my head for a year." (θνητῶν μὲν τέχναις ἀπορούμενος, εἰς δὲ τὸ θεῖον ἐλπίδα πᾶσαν ἔχων προλιπὼν εὔπαιδας Ἀθήνας, ἰάθην ἐλθών, Ἀσκληπιέ, πρὸς τὸ σὸν ἄλσος, ἕλκος ἔχων κεφαλῆς ἐνιαύσιον, ἐν τρισὶ μησίν.) See also Girone 1998, II.1.

64. Ael., *DF* fr. 92 c–e: ὁ δὲ ἀθλίως νόσῳ (περιπνευμονίαν καλοῦσιν Ἀσκληπιαδῶν παῖδες αὐτήν) πιεζόμενος τὰ μὲν πρῶτα ἐδεῖτο τῆς ἀνθρώπων ἰατρικῆς καὶ ἐκείνων ἤρτητο. τῆς τῶν ἰατρῶν ἐπιστήμης βιαιότερον ἦν τὸ νόσημα. ἐπεὶ τοίνυν ὑπὲρ τῶν ἐσχάτων ἐσάλευεν ἤδη, κομίζουσιν αὐτὸν οἱ προσήκοντες ἐς Ἀσκληπιοῦ.

65. Tinker (1983, 108–122) discusses the "motif," as he calls it, of the despair doctors felt about certain patients and their illnesses.

66. *IG* IV² 1 122.55–60=LiDonnici 1995 (B10).

67. *Prorr.* 2.8=9.26 L.; *IG* IV² 1 122.132–133=LiDonnici 1995 (B23); *IG* II² 4514.

68. Dropsy: *Reg. app.* 20=2.496–498 L.; *IG* IV² 1 122.1–6=LiDonnici 1995 (B1). Epilepsy: *Morb.Sacr.* 11=6.380–382 L.; *IG* IV² 1 123.115–117=LiDonnici 1995 (C19).

69. *Morb.Sacr.* 11=6.382 L.: "Whenever the disease [epilepsy] has become chronic, it is no longer curable." (ὁπόταν γὰρ ὁ χρόνος γένηται τῇ νούσῳ οὐκ ἔτι ἰήσιμος γίνεται); also *Aph.* 5.7=4.534 L.

Four • Documeting Asklepios' Arrival in Athens

1. *SEG* 25.226=*IG* II² 4961 4960, associated by Beschi 1967/68. On the introduction of cults to Athens in the fifth century, see Garland 1992; Parker 1996, 152–198. On ancient narratives of cult transfer, see Gebhard 2001. The closest parallel to the account inscribed on the Telemachos monument is an account inscribed on a column in the late third or early second century BC that tells of the founding of a cult of Sarapis on Delos (*IG* XI 4.1299). This account even mentions a legal dispute over the temple of Sarapis (lines 23–38), akin to a land dispute mentioned on the Telemachos monument. On the Sarapis column, see Engelmann 1975.

2. On the integration of Asklepios into the cults of Dionysos Eleuthereus and Eleusinian Demeter, see Chapter 5 below. The only other cult introduced to Athens in the

fifth century that was placed on the Acropolis is that of Pan, in a cave on the Acropolis' northwest shoulder. See Travlos 1971, s.v. "Pan"; Hurwit 1999, 130; Camp 2001, 50. Other cults introduced to Athens in the fifth century include Bendis, Pheme, Artemis Aristoboule, Adrasteia, Meter, Adonis, Sabazius, and possibly Aphrodite Ourania and Aeacus (although the latter two may have arrived in the late sixth century); see Garland 1992; Parker 1996, 152–198.

3. While the earliest inventory (Inventory I, as numbered by Aleshire 1989 = IG II² 1532 fr.b) dates to ca. 350–339/8 BC, it includes dedications from previous years, possibly even from the fifth century.

4. E.g., Ar. Ach. 1030–1032; Pl. Grg. 456b–c; Thucy. 2.47–53.

5. The late manuscripts show more and more invented Ionianisms, and the original texts seem to have been somewhere between Attic and Ionic; see Kühlewein 1894–1902, vol. 1, lxv. My thanks to Kent Rigsby for this reference. Even those treatises that were composed in the Ionic dialect need not have been composed by Ionic Greeks; Hippocrates himself was from Dorian Kos, and Ionic was the dialect of the earliest Greek prose and remained the dialect favored by intellectuals for much of the fifth century; see Longrigg 1993, 32–33. Van der Eijk (1997, 100) proposes that the use of Ionic Greek facilitated a wider reception of ideas since much of the area covered by doctors included Ionic speakers. On Ionic features in early Greek prose, see Dover 1997, 81–95. On Atticisms in On the Art, see Mann 2005, 16. On doctors and rhetorical display, see Jouanna 1999, 75–85. Hippocrates' Life, as reported by Soranus, the Suda, and Tzetzes, all mention Gorgias as one of Hippocrates' teachers.

6. Wickkiser, forthcoming. Those who attribute the importation to plague include Burford 1969, 20; Martin and Metzger 1976, 66–67; Mikalson 1984; Garland 1992, 130–132; Parker 1996, 175–185.

7. Votive reliefs of the late fifth century, as well as later inscriptions and statuettes related to Asklepios, indicate that the god also had a sanctuary in the Agora and perhaps inside the Eleusinion. For discussion and bibliography, see Riethmüller 2005, vol. 2, 11–12; also Lawton, forthcoming.

8. Sources for the importation to Rome are collected in Edelstein and Edelstein 1945, T. 846–854. On the problems of associating Aesculapius, as the Romans called him, with plague in Rome, see also Wickkiser 2003, chs. 7–9.

9. On miasma and plague, see Parker 1983, esp. 257–280.

10. Woodman 1988, 39.

11. Lawton, forthcoming. Woodman 1988, 39–40, with n. 235. For Woodman's discussion of war, plague, and hubris as an established literary convention by the time of Thucydides, see 32–40.

12. Wounds: IG IV² 1 121.95–98 = LiDonnici 1995 (A12); IG IV² 1 122.55–60 = LiDonnici 1995 (B10); IG IV² 1 122.63–68 = LiDonnici 1995 (B12). The latter two were incurred "in some battle" (ἔν τινι μάχαι). Difficulty conceiving: IG IV² 1 122.60–63 = LiDonnici 1995 (B11) (the woman is from Epirus); IG IV² 1 122.82–86 = LiDonnici 1995 (B14) (Troezen has been restored in this inscription as the woman's home); IG IV² 1 122.116–119 = LiDonnici 1995 (B19) (the woman is from Keos); IG IV² 1 122.128–131 = LiDonnici 1995 (B22) (the woman is from Messene).

13. Connolly 1998. Since there is no mention of Telemachos in the Sophocles accounts, scholars reconcile the two traditions by suggesting that Asklepios stopped at Sophocles' *oikia* on his way to the Eleusinion; see, e.g., Clinton 1994a, 25–26. For a list of ancient testimonia and recent bibliography on Sophocles' relationship to Asklepios, see Clinton 1994a, 25 and nn. 26 and 27; and Connolly 1998. Connolly (1998, 10–20) also delves into the history of scholarship on the Sophocles-Asklepios tradition, documenting how opinion has swung from skepticism in the 1880s about the veracity of the reception stories, to a gradual acceptance of them as historical fact due in part to Körte's questionable restorations of key inscriptions in the 1890s. It is a remarkable story of seeing what we wish to see in the evidence.

14. See Lefkowitz 1981, esp. 75–87, for her discussion of the vita of Sophocles.

15. TrGF IV T 1.11.

16. IG II² 1252 + 999; IG II² 1253. Lefkowitz (1981, 84) observes that it would be odd for Sophocles to have been called "Dexion" instead of "Sophocles" in his heroic role since heroes were worshipped under their own names.

17. On the monument on which the paean is inscribed, see Aleshire 1991, 49–59. Other sources also mention a paean by Sophocles to Asklepios: Lucian *Dem.Enc.* 27; Philostr. *VA* 3.17; Philostr.Jun. *Im.* 13.

18. Mitropoulou (1975, 13–42) has assembled a catalogue of most of the fragments, including detailed measurements and photographs. Another fragment was identified later by Beschi and published with photographs in Beschi 1982. See Mitropoulou 1975, 12, for a summary of earlier reconstructions. On the monument's reliefs, see Frel 1975; Ghedini 1980, 15–18; Beschi 1985, 15–19; Beschi 2002; Eliakes 1992–1998. Further bibliography appears in Comella 2002, cat. "Atene 135"; Riethmüller 2005, vol. 1, 241–250, esp. n. 3.

19. For discussion and bibliography regarding the dating, see Beschi 1967/1968, 428–436. The monument may have been erected by Telemachos or his family (although it would be unusual at this time for an individual to erect a monument in his own honor). While this implies a natural bias, it would have been difficult for Telemachos to fabricate and publish such detail about highly public events in a place as prominent as the Asklepieion without recrimination or removal of the monument by the demos.

20. SEG 47.232 is a new edition of lines 1–26 only of SEG 25.226.

21. The most contested readings and restorations in the inscription are at 13–14, as noted by Clinton 1991 21–22: Clinton "δια[κόνος," Dragoumis "διά[κονον," Körte "δ⟨ρ⟩ά[κοντα"; and 15–16: Clinton "Τηλέμαχο[ς] κα[τὰ χρησμ]ός," Kutsch "Τηλ[έ]μαχο[ς κ]α[τὰ χρησμό]ς," Körte "Τηλ[ε]μάχο [ὑπ]α[παντῶντο]ς," Foucart "ἀπ]α[παντῶντο]ς," Wilamowitz "τὸ] ἅ[ρμα ἄγοντο]ς." Regarding διά[κόνος, Clinton (1994a, 23 n. on line 13) states, "There is no doubt about the iota in the 16th stoichos." Parker (1996, 177–178) favors the supplement δράκοντα since snakes "regularly feature in accounts of the introduction of Asclepius." See also Gebhard 2001, 468–471, who argues that Asklepios arrived in the form of a serpent even if the text does not refer to one.

22. Clinton 1994a, 23–24.

23. Clinton 1994a, 24, where Clinton also comments: "The style lacks art, but it serves Telemachos well; it conveniently leaves unsaid what others have contributed in

bringing the cult of Asclepius to Athens." On the establishment and typical components of Greek sanctuaries, see Stengel 1920, 10–31; and Burkert 1985, 84–95.

24. The Telemachos monument does not indicate whether Asklepios came to the center of Athens from a preexisting sanctuary at Zea or directly from Epidauros with Zea as his point of disembarkation. Either is possible. I have opted for the latter interpretation, but my arguments about polis intervention are consistent also with the former, given that even if Athens already had a cult of Asklepios at Zea in 420, it chose to give Asklepios a much more prominent sanctuary on the Acropolis at this time. There is no certain evidence for an Asklepieion at Zea as early as 420; scholars rely on the vague reference to Zea in the Telemachos monument to argue for its early establishment, as discussed by Parker 1996, 181–182, who casts doubts on the supposed early foundation.

25. Agora, inv. no. I 7471, a law about one of Asklepios' annual festivals in Athens, has been restored convincingly to include the word φρουροί, sacred officials whose precise function is not known. For a text and discussion of the law, see Clinton 1994a, 18–21. According to Clinton, φρουροί, otherwise unattested in Attica, were prominent in the cult of Asklepios at Epidauros. Their presence in this Athenian inscription suggests that Athenians deliberately adopted this title and/or that Epidaurian officials participated in the Athenian festival. Clinton argues that, since the Epidauria commemorated Asklepios' arrival in Athens, it is likely that these officials, whether Athenians or Epidaurians, participated in the god's arrival in 420 BC. On the role of φρουροί at Epidauros, see Jeffrey 1966; Clinton 1994a, 20.

26. The perceived minimal role of the state spans the following range. Körte (1896, 1927) argues that the state did not authorize the importation. Aleshire (1989) implies that the state had little involvement since she does not discuss it and since she considers the cult a "private" foundation. Cavanaugh (1996, 47) remarks that the state in the very least must have ratified the importation and allotted the land for the sanctuary. Clinton (1994a) suggests a greater role for the state when he discusses the participation of the cult of Eleusinian Demeter in Asklepios' arrival.

27. E.g., Aleshire 1989, 7; Garland 1992, 128–130; Stafford 2000, 155 with n. 33.

28. For more examples and discussion of the topos, see Garland 1992, 14–22; Gebhard 2001.

29. For the sake of simplicity, I am treating Telemachos as if he were an historical figure. If Telemachos is considered a fictional character, it would presuppose a higher level of state involvement and would thus only strengthen the arguments I am making here. I hope to pursue this aspect at a future date.

30. See, e.g., Rudhardt 1960, 92–93; Garland 1984, 78; Garland 1992, 19; Clinton 1994a, 24–25 and 28; Parker 1996, 180 and 214–217; S. Price 1999, 76–78.

31. Burford (1969, 20), Mikalson (1984), Simms (1985, 284–286), Garland (1992, 130–132), and Parker (1996, 175–185), all speak variously of the interest of the state or of the Athenians, but they trace that interest to the plague. Schlaifer (1940, 240 n. 2) and Cavanaugh (1996, 47) mention state interest in the introduction of the cult but do not comment on the nature of that interest.

32. On the Eleusinion, which has been only partially excavated, see Travlos 1971, s.v. "Eleusinion"; Miles 1998.

33. On the Kerykes, see Clinton 1974, 47–68; Garland 1984, 99–100. The peacemaking Kallias (II) is the grandfather of the Kallias (III) instrumental in bringing Asklepios to Athens; see Chapter 6 below.

34. The best general overview of the cult and its rituals remains Mylonas 1961, although many of his interpretations have been questioned. Kevin Clinton has published extensively on the sanctuary at Eleusis; see the bibliography to this book.

35. On the decrees, which include SEG 21.3–4 and SEG 22.2–3, see Garland 1984, 98. Mylonas (1961, 103–105) argues that the Eleusis sanctuary was reoriented towards Athens at this time, but Jennifer Palinkas (2008), who has restudied the Eleusis propylaia, points out that there is no evidence for such a change. Clinton (1993; 1994b, 161–162) adduces literary and epigraphic evidence suggesting that the Mysteries, and presumably also Eleusis itself, were under Athenian control by the beginning of the seventh century BC.

36. The first artistic representations of Triptolemos date to the mid–sixth century BC; see Shapiro 1989, 67–83. On the significance of Triptolemos to Athens, see Clinton 1994b; Foley 1994, 99–100; Miles 1998, 35–57, esp. 53–56.

37. Growing fifth–century interest in the cult may have been due in part to Demeter's alleged defense of Athens in the Battle of Salamis in 479 BC (Hdt. 8.65). On fifth–century building activity in the sanctuary, see Mylonas 1961, 106–129. Expansions to the sanctuary included the peribolos wall and the area of the east court.

38. Mylonas 1961, 117–124. The most comprehensive analysis of the Telesterion remains Noack 1927.

39. Cavanaugh 1996, 74. IG I³ 78, line 33: hó[τι] ἂν βόλο[νται]. The decree is dated to ca. 460 BC based on letter forms; see Clinton 1974, 10–13; Cavanaugh 1996, 73–74. For this and other sacred laws relating to Eleusis, see also Sokolowski 1969.

40. Bowie 1993, 244; Foley 1994, 144.

41. De Polignac 1995, 85; de Polignac, however, views Athens as an exception to his own model since, in his view, it has no extraurban sanctuary comparable to the Argive Heraion (the rituals of Eleusis, unlike the Heraion, "were reserved solely for initiates"). On processions as defining and articulating space in ancient Greece, see the discussion and bibliography in Graf 1996. On the calendar of the Mysteries, see Deubner 1932, 69–91; Mikalson 1975, 55–61; and Parke 1977, 55–72.

42. On the Lesser Mysteries, see Deubner 1932, 70; Mylonas 1961, 239–243; and Parke 1977, 122–124. According to Athenian tradition, this festival was introduced to initiate Herakles, a foreigner, into the Mysteries (Schol. ad Ar. Pl. 1013; Diod.Sic. 4.14; Plut. Thes. 30), much as Asklepios' arrival explains the integration of the Epidauria (discussed in Chapter 5 below) into the Greater Mysteries.

43. See Clinton 1994a, 18–19 and 29, citing Agora inv. no. I 7471, which mentions priests of Demeter in relation to the Epidauria.

44. Storage of ritual objects in the Eleusinion: Syll.³ 885; sacrifices: Mylonas 1961, 250–251.

45. Pausanias' narrative suggests that the Epidauria were founded at the time of Asklepios' arrival in Athens, which accords with the claim of the Telemachos monument that Asklepios arrived while the Mysteries were underway. A sacred law from the Athe-

nian Agora dating to 410–404 BC makes reference to the Epidauria within the context of the Mysteries (Agora inv. no. I 7471, mentioned above); see Clinton 1994a, 27. It is uncertain which day of the Mysteries coincides with the Epidauria; see Mikalson 1975, 56.

46. Clinton 1994a, 24–25.

47. On the Epidauria, see Deubner 1932, 73; Parke 1977, 63–65; Parker 2005, 462 s.v. "Asklpieia"; also Clinton 1994a, 29, who argues that the Epidauria included a procession reenacting Asklepios' arrival.

48. Clinton (1994a, 28–34) argues that the land dispute is indicative of a larger friction between Telemachos and the Kerykes: the latter had wanted to align Asklepios more closely with the cult of Demeter by housing him nearer the Eleusinion, and they grew angry when Telemachos moved Asklepios to the Acropolis.

49. In Chapter 6, I suggest a reason why the Kerykes may have wanted to remove Asklepios in 418 BC.

50. Thucy. 2.15.3–6.

51. See Travlos 1971, s.v. "Athena Nike" and "Erechtheion"; Hurwit 1999, 200–215, and app. C.13–15 for ancient sources and bibliography.

52. On the Odeion, see Hurwit 1999, 216–217, and app. C.19 for ancient sources and bibliography. Hurwit (1999, 217) suggests that the theater was also altered at this time: "It is difficult to believe that the Periklean program would have created so vast a building as the Odeion without paying at least some attention to the Theater next door, and there is the possibility of some kind of Periklean refitting."

53. On the topography and architectural development of the sanctuary, see Travlos 1971, s.v. "Asklepieion"; Aleshire 1989, 21–36; Hurwit 1999, 219–221, with app. C.20 for ancient sources and bibliography; Riethmüller 2005, vol. 1, 241–273; Melfi 2007, 313–409. Although the predominant view is that the sanctuary ultimately included the western terrace, with its Ionic banqueting hall, this matter is still under debate. Riethmüller (1999, 156–178) for example, argues that the sanctuary was confined to the eastern terrace (a stretch of some 55 m); see Riethmuller 1999, 120 with nn. 14–11 for bibliography. For critique of Riethmüller's arguments, see Lefantzis and Jensen, forthcoming.

54. Beschi 1967/1968, 386–397. On the Pelargikon, see Travlos 1971, s.v. "Akropolis"; Camp 1984; Hurwit 1999, 78. Thucy. 2.17 describes how people forced to flee the Attic countryside in the early years of the Peloponnesian War sought refuge within the Pelargikon despite the fact that residence within it was forbidden by a curse and cautioned against by the oracle at Delphi.

55. Cavanaugh (1996, 29–72) provides an extensive summary of scholarship on the debate over the date of this decree. Of the sixty-seven sources she lists and their proposed dates, plus her own suggested date, only eighteen include a date or date range that falls after 420 BC and the arrival of Asklepios. Many of these eighteen have followed the assumptions of Körte (1896, 1927) that the establishment of the Asklepieion prompted the rider and that the cult thus arrived without state authorization; see Cavanaugh 55–59. As Cavanaugh (47) remarks, however, "The idea that the Asklepieion could be established without the consent of the Athenian demos is unthinkable." In the very least, it is unlikely. Some of the scholars she lists as proponents of a post-420 date, like Clinton (1974), have subsequently favored an earlier date; cf. Clinton 1994a, 32 with n. 65. Cavanaugh's own

arguments against a date post-422/21 BC, based on publication at that time of a decree (IG I³ 391) reflecting changes to IG I³ 78, are persuasive.

56. IG I³ 78, lines 54–59: "The King (Archon) shall delimit the sanctuaries in the Pelargikon, and in the future altars shall not be erected in the Pelargikon without the consent of the Boule and the People, nor shall (anyone) cut stones out of the Pelargikon, or remove soil or stones. If anyone transgresses any of these regulations, he shall be fined five hundred drachmas and impeached by the King (Archon) before the Boule." Translated by C.W. Fornara (1983).

57. On the path of the Pelargikon, see Hurwit 1999, 78, with bibliography at n. 42.

58. Robert Schlaifer (1940, 240 n. 2) comments, "The mere granting by the state of permission to build on so well situated a site, indicate[s] that the state was seriously interested in the cult from the beginning." Simms (1985, 285, following Schlaifer) regards the location of the cult on the Acropolis ("the religious center of the city") as indicative of the state's interest in the cult. Simms, however, attributes the importation of the cult to plague.

Five • Asklepios and the Topography of Athenian Cult

1. On the Athenian calendar, see Deubner 1932; Mikalson 1975; Parke 1977; Bruit Zaidman and Schmitt Pantel 1992, 102–107; S. Price 1999, 28–30. Although aspects of the Attic festival calendar antedate the Ionian migration, as discussed by Burkert (1992b, 543), the polis would have controlled additions to the calendar.

2. Water was used in Asklepieia for ritual bathing and also for practical matters like drinking. However, the spring on the eastern terrace of the Asklepieion was not the only water source on the Acropolis, much less in Athens. It is unlikely, therefore, that this spring was the definitive factor in locating the sanctuary. On Athenian water sources, see Camp 1977.

3. On the Acropolis as a "text," see Hurwit 1999, 228–232. In "The Wobbling Pivot," J.Z. Smith (1978, 88–103) has stressed the importance of the periphery as well as the center (championed by Mircea Eliade) to studies of sacred space.

4. Hurwit 1999, 232.

5. On the history, mythology, and archaeology of the Acropolis from the Neolithic to the modern periods, see Hurwit 1999 and Holtzmann 2003. The earliest literary account of Athena's victory over Poseidon is Hdt. 8.55. According to Thucydides (2.15.3–6), Athens' early inhabitants lived on the Acropolis.

6. On the accommodation of Mycenaean remains, see Hurwit 1999, 159–160. Paus. 1.24.5 describes the Parthenon pediments; see also Binder 1984; Palagia 1993.

7. Hurwit 1999, 228–232.

8. The date of the battle at Eurymedon, as with most dates of Thucydides' *pentekontaetia* (Thucy. 1.89–118) is also disputed. For chronologies, see Gomme 1945–1981, vol. 1, pp. 394, 397, 408; Badian 1993; Pritchett 1995. The historicity of the Peace of Kallias has been disputed since the fourth century BC; on the debate and relevant bibliography, see Badian 1987.

9. For discussion, ancient sources, and bibliography on the architecture, construction, and symbolism of the Parthenon, see Hurwit 1999, esp. app. C.3; and Holtzmann 2003. On the financing of the Periklean building program and Athens' own ambivalent reactions to the financing, see Kallet 1998.

10. The tribute lists record not the full tribute but the first fruits, or one-sixtieth of the total tribute, paid by Athens' subject-allies.

11. IG I³ 14, 40, 46, 48. For additional signs of Athenian imperialism on the Acropolis, see Shear 2001, 17–18, 724–768.

12. Hurwit (1999, 54) addresses the issue of literacy in regard to the numerous inscriptions on the Acropolis. He suggests that "the principal of publication may have mattered more than the actual practice of reading" and that the formulaic nature of most of the inscriptions enabled them to be interpreted even by those with little ability to read. Hedrick (1994, 174) asserts that inscriptions served the democracy as mnemonic devices of "what everyone already knows." However, Sickinger (1999, 78) adduces a phrase appearing on some fifth-century inscriptions, "for whoever wishes to scrutinize" (εἰδέναι τοι βουλομένοι e.g., IG I³ 84), to demonstrate that inscriptions were erected, at least in part, to be read and examined. How many Athenians could read them remains uncertain.

13. Shear 2001 offers a comprehensive, diachronic study of the history, composition, and topography of the festival. For the early history of the festival and description of its rituals, see Deubner 1932, 22–35; and Parke 1977, 33–50. On the democratic and imperial implications of the Panathenaia in the Periklean period, see Shapiro 1996.

14. Erythrai, for instance, was required to bring an offering, probably of grain, to the festival (IG I³ 14). The date of this decree is disputed, but it falls somewhere between 470 and 450 BC based on letter forms; see ML 40. Brea, an Athenian colony, was required to send a cow and suit of armor (IG I³ 46). The date of this decree is also disputed; see ML 49. Another decree, possibly from the 440s BC, requires certain cities of the empire to send a cow and panoply (IG I³ 34); see ML 46. On participation by Athenian allies and colonists, see Shear 2001, 139–143.

15. The tribute quota lists from 450, 446, and 434 BC indicate changes in the amount of tribute, and therefore reassessment. These same years coincide with celebration of the Greater Panathenaia; see ML 39. Specific stipulations regarding reassessment in years of the Greater Panathenaia appear also in IG I³ 71.

16. The procession wound from the Dipylon Gate through the Agora, by the Eleusinion, and up to the Acropolis, as attested by Thucy. 6.56–57; Xen. Eq.Mag. 3.2; Dem. 34.39; Schol. ad Ar. Eq. 566; Paus. 1.2.14, 1.29.1; Philostr. VS 2.1.5. See also Shear 2001. On the wheeled ship as symbol of naval empire, see Shapiro 1996, 217. Shear (143–154, 163–164), however, cautions that there is no explicit evidence for a ship in the procession before the second century AD. Both IG I³ 14 and IG I³ 46 were found on the Acropolis in the area of the Erechtheum; see ML 40, 49.

17. On the dedication and storage of the panoplies given to Athens by her colonies and allies, see Hurwit 1999, 60; and Shear 2001, 187–195. Gold crowns dedicated at the Greater Panathenaia are also listed in Athena's inventories beginning in 400/399 BC (IG II² 1385.17–18); see Shear 2001, 195–200. Moreover, Athena had become a prominent

symbol of Athenian empire outside Athens. League-cults of "Athena, Ruler of Athens" (Ἀθηνῶν μεδέουσα) spread to such places as Kos and Samos in the fifth century; see Barron 1964 and Parker 1996, 144 with n. 92.

18. Travlos 1971 (s.v. "Athena Nike") argues for a period of construction from 427 to 424 BC; Mark 1993 argues for the period 424/3–418 BC. For further bibliography on the dating dispute, see Schultz 2001, 1 n. 2. See also Hurwit 1999, app. C.14, for ancient sources.

19. Stewart 1985; Hurwit 1999, 211–213. The friezes of Greeks fighting Greeks were situated on the north and west sides of the temple and thus were visible to those ascending the Acropolis. Schultz 2001 situates the temple's references to Nike within the larger context of Athenian victory monuments.

20. The date when construction began (often given as 421 BC) is conjectural, based on an assumption that only with the Peace of Nicias would there have been resources to build such an elaborate structure; see Hurwit 1999, 206, and app. C.13 for ancient sources and bibliography. On integration of the Persian invasion into the Erechtheus myth, see Cook 1995, esp. 134 n. 23.

21. The name Eleuthereus is a reference to Eleutherai, a town on the northern border of Attica whence Dionysos Eleuthereus came to Athens. On Dionysos at Eleusis, see Mylonas 1960; Graf 1974, 40–78; Clinton 1992, 65–67, 123–125.

22. Soph. Ant. 1119–1121: μέδεις δὲ παγκοίνοις Ἐλευσινίας Δηοῦς ἐν κόλποις.

23. Clinton 1992, 123–125.

24. Regarding the prominence of the Eleusinian Dionysia, Clinton (1992, 124) states, "The Dionysia at Eleusis were certainly one of the major celebrations of the Rural Dionysia; indeed they may have been the most renowned such festival in Attica." Another Eleusinian festival, the Haloa, was celebrated in honor of Demeter, and, according to later sources, included Dionysos. However, skepticism has been cast on his presence in this festival, especially for the Classical period; see Brumfield 1981, 104–131. On the inscriptions mentioning the Eleusinian Dionysia, see also Pickard-Cambridge 1968, 47–48.

25. Iakchos' presence in the procession is attested by Hdt. 8.65 and Ar. Ran. 316–317. IG II² 1078 (third century AD) mentions his reception; see also Clinton 1988, 70. Clinton (1992, 66) argues that the god Iakchos developed as a personification of the cry "iakche" voiced during the Mysteries.

26. Clinton (1992, 66) tentatively identifies this as the earliest use of Iakchos in reference to Dionysos. For other ancient sources that interchange or confuse the names, see Clinton 1992, 66 with nn. 22 and 23.

27. One Dionysiac element of the Mysteries was that after reaching Eleusis worshippers took part in all-night revelry (παννυχίς). On other Dionysiac aspects of the procession to Eleusis, see Graf 1974, 55–58.

28. See Burkert 1987, 21–22.

29. On ties between Dionysos and Demeter, see Detienne 1989, 37–38. Many other gods also gave civilizing gifts to humans, like Athena and Asklepios.

30. At Thebes, the sanctuary of Demeter Thesmophoros was located at the house of Kadmos (Paus. 9.16.5) where Semele, the mother of Dionysos, was said to have been buried; see Schachter 1981–, vol. 1, p. 166. Pind. Isth. 7.3–5 describes Dionysos as the

partner of cymbal-sounding Demeter (χαλκοκρότου πάρεδρον Δαμάτερος). As Privitera (1982, ad loc.) points out, however, Pindar's use of πάρεδρος does not always imply a cultic association. Admittedly, the lack of evidence elsewhere may be misleading. Parker's comments (1988) on the cults of Demeter and Dionysos at Sparta are instructive: noting that there is little evidence for Dionysos relative to Demeter, Parker cautions that the situation in Sparta may have derived more from historical factors than regional traditions. Demeter and Dionysos appear together in works of visual art outside Attica, but mainly in the farther reaches of the Greek world (e.g., Kerch on the north coast of the Black Sea, and Magna Graecia).

31. On the topography of the south slope, see Wycherley 1978, 179–185; Aleshire 1989, 21–36. The identification of the sanctuaries to the west of the Asklepieion is debated; see S. Walker 1979.

32. In John Travlos' plan of the Asklepieion (Travlos 1971, fig. 171), it is evident that the paving of the eastern terrace is clipped at its southeastern edge to accommodate the curve of the cavea.

33. On the establishment of the Asklepieia, see Mikalson 1998, 37. Parke (1977, 186) speculates that the festival marks the date of the consecration of Asklepios' sanctuary, which may have occurred in March 419 (the first City Dionysia after Asklepios' arrival). On its rituals, see Deubner 1932, 142; Parke 1977, 135; Parker 2005, 462, s.v. "Asklepieia." IG II² 1496 records the revenue received by the state for the sale of the skins of animals used at various sacrifices and festivals from 334–330 BC. The Asklepieia appears among them, and the amount of revenue is high enough to suggest large numbers of animals, probably for sacrifice. IG II² 974 (second century BC) mentions an all-night celebration and the sacrifice of a bull.

34. The best description of a proagon is that to the Lenaia in Pl. Symp. 194b.

35. Parke 1977, 135. Parke explains the connection between Asklepios and Dionysos through Sophocles, whom some credit with welcoming Asklepios to Athens, as discussed in Chapter 4 above. The many problems with this tradition, however, render arguments based on it problematic.

36. Soph. Phil. 1333–1334. Mitchell-Boyask (2007) discusses how the topography of the south slope sanctuaries may have influenced the production of the Philoktetes. Aristophanes' Ploutos is also evocative of the topography of the Acropolis (although we do not know if this play was performed in the Theater of Dionysos): it describes a visit to a sanctuary of Asklepios, with the final scene being an elaborate procession engineered to reinstall Wealth on the Acropolis where once he guarded Athena's treasury (1191–1193). Within a century of Asklepios' arrival, the cults of Asklepios and Dionysos Eleuthereus were even more closely integrated: in 328, a priest of Asklepios named Androkles was honored for his role as priest of Asklepios and also for his care of the Theater of Dionysos (IG II² 354). The decree was awarded in the month Elaphebolion, the same month as the City Dionysia and Asklepieia. For discussion of the decree, see Schwenk 1985, no. 54.

37. Wiles 1997, 43. Early studies of theater that promote a mode of Epidaurian or "Apollonian" influence on Athens' theater include Fiechter 1930–1950; Pickard-Cambridge 1968; also Travlos 1971. Wiles (44) rejects this view: "The Apolline model is seductive, and we must be cautious of it." See also Rehm 2002, 39–41. On the change from rectangular

to circular theaters, see von Gerkan and Müller-Wiener 1961; Burford 1969, 75–76; Käppel 1989.

38. Wiles 1997, 43–44. The date of the stone theater in Athens is uncertain, but evidence points to the late fourth century; see Tomlinson 1983, 87. A reference in Pl. *Ion* 530a to rhapsodic and unspecified other musical competitions (καὶ τῆς ἄλλης γε μουσικῆς) at Epidauros presumably in the fifth century suggests that an earlier theater existed, but we have no evidence for its location, construction, or design.

39. By the fifth century, we see the metaphor of an ailing state in other genres of poetry and in prose: Solon 4.17; Thgn. 39–40, 1133–1134; Pind. *Pyth.* 4.270–271; Hdt. 3.76.2, 3.127.1, 7.148.3; Thucy. 6.14; Ar. *Vesp.* 650–651. See also Brock 2000; Kosak 2000. On the metaphor in Thucydides, see Kallet 1999.

40. Mikalson 1998, 42–44. Mikalson lists fourth-century evidence for Asklepios as a healer of the body politic.

41. On Dionysiac symbols and the god's healing role, see Burkert 1983, 58–72; Detienne 1989, 27–41.

42. Athen. *Deip.* 1.22, 2.36; Hesych. s.v. "παιώνιος." Athena, too, received the epithet Παιωνία (Paus. 1.2.5). Parker (1983, 288 n. 36) believes that Dionysos' title "doctor" is due to the therapeutic value of wine, and, citing Dodds, he remarks that "in the historical period . . . there is little evidence for a healing Dionysus."

43. Parke (1977, 135) comments: "There is no usual connection between him [Asklepios] and Dionysus."

44. See Wiles 1997 for a spatial analysis of the sanctuary of Dionysos and of the visual axis uniting the sanctuary and the Acropolis. Column drums from an earlier Parthenon were built into the fortification wall along the north side of the Acropolis in the fifth century BC, a visual shorthand for the Parthenon to those standing to the north of the Acropolis, and a reminder of the Persian destruction.

45. Rehm 2002, 37. On the composition and size of the audience, see Winkler 1990; Ley 1991, 33–34; Wiles 1997, 51. Estimates of the size of the audience vary. According to Pl. *Symp.* 175e, the fifth-century audience of the Theater of Dionysos was 30,000.

46. See Wiles 1997, 54–55; Hurwit 1999, 216–218, and app. C.19 for sources and bibliography.

47. The Odeion that stood when these men wrote was not the fifth-century Odeion but a later rebuilding. The Athenians burned the earlier Odeion in 86 BC to preempt Sulla's pillaging of it; see Hurwit 1999, 217. Debates about the building's history continue; see Robkin 1979; M.C. Miller 1997, 218–242. Resemblances between Persian architecture, particularly the Hall of 100 Columns at Persepolis, and the Odeion are discussed by Broneer 1943; von Gall 1977; Root 1985 (whose focus is a comparison of the Parthenon frieze and the Apadana reliefs at Persepolis); Nielsen 1999, 48–49.

48. Shear (2001, 770–772) argues that construction of the Odeion added a new dimension to the Kerameikos—Agora—Acropolis axis that had previously dominated the Greater Panathenaia.

49. The length of the festival is discussed by Mikalson 1975, 123–129. During the Peloponnesian War, the festival was reduced to four days. On the events of the City Dio-

nysia, and for ancient sources, see Deubner 1932, 138–142; Pickard-Cambridge 1968, 57–125; Parke 1977, 125–135; Goldhill 1990.

50. Winkler 1990; Goldhill 1990.

51. On the ritual of the Athenian public funeral, see Loraux 1986.

52. The *Acharnians* was produced at the Lenaia, the other major festival of Dionysos in Athens. Dikaiopolis is able to speak freely to the audience because he is at the Lenaia rather than the City Dionysia.

53. Schol. ad Ar. Ach. 504. Ar. Ach. 504–506: Αὐτοὶ γάρ ἐσμεν οὑπὶ Ληναίῳ τ' ἀγών, | κοὔπω ξένοι πάρεισιν· οὔτε γὰρ φόροι | ἥκουσιν οὔτ' ἐκ τῶν πόλεων οἱ ξύμμαχοι ("For now we are by ourselves at the Lenaia; strangers are not yet present. Neither the tribute nor representatives from the allied cities have yet arrived.") It is generally believed that Athens fixed this date for tribute payment because the City Dionysia coincided with the re-opening of the sailing season; boats carrying tribute to Athens could not sail during winter storms. The arrival of the allies by sea bringing tribute echoes Dionysos' arrival by ship bringing good things, like viticulture, to the city.

54. Rehm (2002, 53) proposes that the practice of parading and laying out tribute may have begun with the transfer of the Delian League treasury to Athens in 454 BC.

55. On these centripetal processions, see Graf 1996, 57–59. Graf considers the procession of the City Dionysia an inversion of the Panathenaic procession because it terminates on the south slope of the Acropolis, "a place for non-civic cults." But at least some of the cults on the south slope, especially that of Dionysos, were very much civic cults. On other similarities between these processions, see Seaford 1994, 248–249.

56. Sourvinou-Inwood (1994) points to further rituals of both festivals that were articulated by the polis as a whole rather than by subdivisions, such as phratries, characteristic of other Athenian festivals.

57. This decree was inscribed, along with a second decree, in 423 BC. The date of the first decree is disputed but falls within the first half of the 420s BC; see ML 65.

58. Thucy. 4.118; 5.23. The peace was also to be renewed at the Hyakinthia in Sparta.

59. Benedum 1986.

60. Benedum 1986, 154–157; also Edelstein and Edelstein 1945, vol. 2, 127–128; Garland 1992, 124. Demeter's gift of a better afterlife is described in the *Homeric Hymn to Demeter* 480–489; Isoc. 4.4.28; Pind. fr. 137a; Soph. fr. 837 Radt.

61. Parker 1996, 180 n. 96.

62. More intriguing but also problematic is Demeter's role as Κουροτρόφος, or nurturer of children, a function related to health. According to Pausanias, sanctuaries of Ge Kourotrophos and Demeter Chloe stood on the slopes of the Acropolis (Paus. 1.22.3). These sanctuaries have not yet been identified nor do we know their date, but Pausanias' description suggests that they lay near the Asklepieion. If so, then Asklepios could have been associated with the kourotrophos aspects of Demeter and Ge via spatial and ritual proximity. On Demeter Chloe and Ge Kourotrophos, see Pauly-Wissowa, s.v. "Demeter" (§28) and "Gaia"; T.H. Price 1978, esp. 101–132 on Attica.

63. For the date of this decree and its rider concerning sanctuaries within the Pelargikon, see Chapter 4 above.

64. For further discussion of this decree and of its date, see Chapter 4 above.

65. Parker 1996, 143; see also Cavanaugh 1996, xiii, for a similar interpretation. Although the influence and prestige of the Eleusinian cult could have been a basis in its own right for making such demands, it is probably not coincidental that the decree came about at a time of Athenian confidence in its hegemony.

66. Parker 1996, 144.

67. Schol. ad Ar. Eq. 566.

68. Syll.³ 885.16. See also Parke 1977, 60. The Athenian demos and boule also authorized construction, in 422/21, of a bridge over a shallow salt-water pond (one of the Rheitoi) that initiates had to cross when traveling between Athens and Eleusis. The inscribed decree authorizing this bridge (IG I³ 79) was crowned by a relief depicting Athena and Demeter, along with Kore and a young male, perhaps Ploutos. See Mark 1993, 77, 88; Lawton 1995, 82–83, no. 3, pl. 2; Lawton, forthcoming.

69. Recently, e.g., Seaford 1994, 243–251; Anderson 2003, 178–194.

Six • Asklepios and Athenian Empire

1. Jameson 1994, 76. Athenian interest in the Saronic Gulf seems to extend even into the sixth century BC, when Athens was part of an amphictionic alliance based at the sanctuary of Poseidon in Kalauria (Strabo 8.6.14 [C 374]). The amphictiony included Hermione, Epidauros, Aegina, Nauplia, Prasiai, and Boeotian Orchomenos. Kalauria, Aegina, and Epidauros are all on the Saronic Gulf, and Hermione is only slightly beyond, lying farther south along the coast of the Akte peninsula facing the island Hydra.

2. Jameson 1994, 76.

3. The other territories attacked were Halieis, Hermione, and Troezen. For earlier Athenian relations with Halieis and Hermione, see Gomme 1945–1981, vol. 1, p. 311, 367.

4. Gomme 1945–1981, vol. 3, p. 495, suggests that Epidauros was successful in resisting these attacks because Athens was involved in too many theaters of warfare at the time.

5. Thucy. 5.53.1: "During the same summer, war broke out between the Epidaurians and Argives. The alleged reason for this was a sacrifice to Apollo Pythaeus that the Epidaurians were required to send, but were not sending. The Argives were in control of this sanctuary. Aside from this cause, it seemed best to Alcibiades and the Argives to acquire Epidauros if they could in order both to keep Corinth quiet and to provide a shorter route for Athenians bringing help (to Argos) via Aegina, rather than sailing all the way around Skyllaion." (τοῦ δ'αὐτοῦ θέρους Ἐπιδαυρίοις καὶ Ἀργείοις πόλεμος ἐγένετο, προφάσει μὲν περὶ τοῦ θύματος τοῦ Ἀπόλλωνος τοῦ Πυθαέως, ὃ δέον ἀπαγαγεῖν οὐκ ἀπέπεμπον ὑπὲρ βοταμίων Ἐπιδαύριοι [κυριώτατοι δὲ τοῦ ἱεροῦ ἦσαν Ἀργεῖοι]· ἐδόκει δὲ καὶ ἄνευ τῆς αἰτίας τὴν Ἐπίδαυρον τῷ τε Ἀλκιβιάδῃ καὶ τοῖς Ἀργείοις προσβαλεῖν, ἢν δύνωνται, τῆς τε Κορίνθου ἕνεκα ἡσυχίας καὶ ἐκ τῆς Αἰγίνης βραχυτέραν ἔσεσθαι τὴν βοήθειαν ἢ Σκύλλαιον περιπλεῖν τοῖς Ἀθηναίοις.) Corinth had proved troublesome to Athens for many years. Its poor relations with Corcyra, according to Thucy. 1.24–55, had been a major factor triggering the Peloponnesian War. Even in 421 BC, after the conclusion of the Peace

of Nicias, Corinth tried to engineer a defensive alliance of Greek states that would refuse to ally with Athens or Sparta (Thucy. 5.27–32).

6. That same summer, Alcibiades tried unsuccessfully to build a fort at Achaean Rhion on the mouth of the Gulf of Corinth just across from Naupaktos, then held by Athens (Thucy. 5.52). With a military presence at Rhion as well as Naupaktos, Athens would effectively have gained control of the gulf, as noted by Gomme 1945–1981, vol. 4, p. 70. This attempt is another indication of Athenian desire to control sea as well as land routes to and from the Peloponnese.

7. Gomme 1945–1981, vol. 4, p. 77, notes that Athens did not disclaim responsibility for the Spartan advance. Certain Athenians, like Alcibiades, were clearly interested in resuming war with Sparta, and therefore may have let the Spartans advance in order to have an excuse to return to war with them.

8. According to Polyaenus 3.9.48, the Athenian general Iphikrates plundered Epidauros in 372 BC. It is not clear from his account, however, why Iphikrates was at Epidauros other than to pillage. Beginning ca. 390 BC, Athenian craftsmen helped with the fourth-century construction efforts at the Epidaurian Asklepieion. Their names are listed on building accounts published in the sanctuary (IG IV² 1 102–120); see Burford 1969. As Avalos (1995, 93–98) has argued, participation of Athenian craftsmen in work at this panhellenic sanctuary is not necessarily indicative of foreign relations between Athens and Epidauros. Dillon (1997) shows that panhellenic sanctuaries often remained accessible even to individuals coming from enemy states.

9. Athens' frequent attempts to overtake the Megarid confirm its desire to control the land corridor between Attica and the Peloponnese. On the importance of the Megarid to both Athens and the Peloponnese during the war, see Thucy. 2.93, 4.66–69. Jameson (1994, 80–81) comments, "The fighting that marked the end of Spartan dominance [in the fourth century BC] showed the strategic importance of the states on and around the Isthmos of Corinth for any power intending to control both central and southern Greece."

10. Burford 1969.

11. Gomme 1945–1981, vol. 2, p. 163.

12. Epidauros assisted Corinth in the Corcyrean affair and supported the Megarian revolt against Athens; cf. Thucy. 1.27.2, 1.114.1.

13. Thucy. 1.23.6: "But I believe the truest cause—and the least apparent—was that the Athenians were becoming greater, and the Lacedaimonians grew afraid, which drove them to war." (τὴν μὲν γὰρ ἀληθεστάτην πρόφασιν, ἀφανεστάτην δὲ λόγῳ, τοὺς Ἀθηναίους ἡγοῦμαι μεγάλους γιγνομένους καὶ φόβον παρέχοντας τοῖς Λακεδαιμονίοις ἀναγκάσαι ἐς τὸ πολεμεῖν.) Cf. also Thucy. 1.88, 1.139.3, 2.8.4.

14. Thucy. 5.26.1–2: "Up until this point [404 BC], the war lasted 27 years altogether. And if anyone should not think it right to include the intervening truce in that war, they will not judge correctly. For let them assess the deeds as they have been recounted and they will find that such a situation—in which everything agreed on had neither been given back nor received—cannot be judged a peace." (ἔτη δὲ ἐς τοῦτο τὰ ξύμπαντα ἐγένετο τῷ πολέμῳ ἑπτὰ καὶ εἴκοσι. καὶ τὴν διὰ μέσου ξύμβασιν εἴ τις μὴ ἀξιώσει πόλεμον νομίζειν, οὐκ ὀρθῶς δικαιώσει. τοῖς [τε] γὰρ ἔργοις ὡς διῄρηται ἀθρείτω, καὶ

εὑρήσει οὐκ εἰκὸς ὃν εἰρήνην αὐτὴν κριθῆναι, ἐν ᾗ οὔτε ἀπέδοσαν πάντα οὔτ᾽ ἀπεδέξαντο ἃ ξυνέθεντο.)

15. A copy of the treaty was erected near the Theater of Dionysos in Athens (IG I³ 83).

16. Extensive bibliography on Peisistratos and his contributions appears in Parker 1996, 67–101. But Parker (1996, 69) cautions: "The religious chronology of the [sixth century] is thus a concertina, which if squeezed brings all the relevant events within the Peisistratid period, if stretched puts almost all outside. In the name of caution—and perhaps even of truth—one should speak more generally of 'the sixth century expansion' rather than more specifically of 'Peisistratean religious policy.'" See also Osborne 1994, who argues that Athens manipulated cults for political reasons long before Peisistratos.

17. E.g., Parker 1996, 187: "What is truly striking is the extent to which the new foundations of the fifth century reflect in one way or another its great historical centerpiece, the struggle against Persia."

18. On these and other cult developments in the wake of the Persian War, see Parker 1996, 152–198.

19. On Theseus and Athens, see Garland 1992, 82–98; H.J. Walker 1995; Calame 1996. On the Theseus legend, see also the collection of essays in Ward et al. 1970.

20. The five figures Theseus encountered were Sinis (on the Isthmus), Krommyon (on the border of Corinth and Megara), Skiron (at Megara), Kerkyron (near Eleusis), and Procrustes (between Eleusis and Athens).

21. On Theseus in Attic vase painting and sculpture, see Neils 1987. For the date when these labors began to appear, see Neils 1987, 36–37. The labors also appear on the late Archaic Athenian treasury at Delphi and on the Hephaestaeon in Athens (ca. 450 BC). For Theseus in Greek tragedy, see Mills 1997.

22. While the importance of the Corinthiad would become increasingly apparent during the Peloponnesian War, by the sixth century Athens already recognized the strategic importance of the Megarid (on major land routes into Attica, Boeotia, and the Peloponnese) and had fought Megara over control of Salamis: Hdt. 1.59; Arist. Ath.Pol. 14, 17; Plu. Solon 8; Diog.Laert. 1.47. Moreover, since Athenian tradition posited the Isthmus as the frontier between Ionia and the Peloponnese, and Megara as part of Ionia, Athens believed Megara should be under its control: Pl. Crit. 110d; Hdt. 5.76; Strabo 3.5.5 (C 171), 9.1.5 (C 392); Paus. 1.39.4. Eleusis, also in the Megarid, had long since been under Attic influence; see Osborne 1994, 148–154, for archaeological evidence indicating cultural uniformity between Athens and Eleusis since at least the Dark Age.

23. The earliest literary evidence for the encounter with Periphetes is Augustan (Diod. Sic. 4.59; also mentioned in Plut. Thes. 1.2; ps-Apollod. 3.15). It may appear on a late Archaic metope of the Athenian treasury at Delphi and on a mid-fifth-century metope of the Hephaestaeon in Athens, but as Nilsson (1951, 54) comments, "The interpretation is not at all evident." See also Neils 1987, 48 and 127. Neils (1987, 122 and 127) points out that the Periphetes episode is unknown in vase painting, with one unlikely exception.

24. H.J. Walker 1995, 42, following Calame 1996, 422.

25. The date is disputed. An Athenian inscription recording the accounts of the treasurers of the other gods for 429/8 BC includes an entry for Bendis (IG I³ 383.143), but the

earliest reliable evidence for a temple of Bendis is Xen. *Hell.* 2.4.11, which concerns events in 404/3 BC. See Planeaux 2000–2001 for bibliography and discussion of the date of Bendis' entry.

26. Nilsson 1951, 46; also Garland 1992, 112. Planeaux 2000–2001 argues that Bendis arrived in Athens in response also to the plague. Planeaux considers this a reason for the appeal of the goddess to the citizens at large. The date of Bendis' entry, if 429/8 BC, is much more compelling than Asklepios' in relation to the plague of 431 BC, but Planeaux's arguments for a link between Bendis and healing are tenuous. Deloptes, Bendis' male consort, whom Planeaux associates iconographically with Asklepios, is too poorly attested in art to render convincing any strong connection between him and Asklepios (there is only one depiction of him that is certain; see *LIMC* s.v. "Deloptes," no. 1).

27. Nilsson 1951, 33; Garland 1992, 115. Garland concludes his study by cautioning, "Yet the treatment of Athenian religion *merely* as an extension of her political and social aspirations, and to extrapolate from it *merely* a coded commentary on Athens' relationship with herself and the outside world, is to miss half the point, because religion was not an epiphenomenon of a state's temporal aspirations" (1992, 172, emphasis Garland's).

28. Clinton (1994a, 30–31) raises this point. As further indication of cooperation between Epidauros and the Kerykes, he also mentions a fourth-century priest of Asklepios at Zea who was a member of the Kerykes. His conclusions as to the importance of Epidauros to Athens differ from my own, however. He suggests that Asklepios was imported from Epidauros and incorporated into the Eleusinian Mysteries to boost Demeter's waning popularity at Athens.

29. Clinton 1994a, 18.

30. Garland (1992, 126) suggests that the support of Athens and Eleusis were key to catapulting the cult of Asklepios to panhellenic fame. Athens' role in this fame should not be overstated, however. The cult at Epidauros was rapidly acquiring a panhellenic following before Asklepios reached Athens.

31. Garland 1992, 122.

32. Thucy. 5.53: ἐδόκει δὲ . . . τὴν Ἐπίδαυρον τῷ Ἀλκιβιάδῃ καὶ τοῖς Ἀργείοις προσλαβεῖν, ἢν δύνωνται.

33. Gomme (1945–1981, vol. 4, p. 70) comments, "It was a grandiose scheme for an Athenian general at the head of a mainly Peloponnesian army to march through the Peloponnese, cocking a snook at Sparta when her reputation was at its lowest."

34. On Kallias, see J.K. Davies 1971, 254–269; Clinton 1974, 49–50.

35. Clinton 1994a, 30.

36. See also Nilsson 1951, 27–28, who argues that Peisistratos rather than Solon brought Salamis under Athenian control.

37. Feeney 1998, 120. No one would deny, however, that rituals have the capacity for meaning and that we can recover some of that meaning by analysis of the context and conventions (literary, ritual, etc.) surrounding them. For a judicious assessment of the challenges and possibilities of "reading" rituals in Athens, see Connor 1987.

38. Woodman 1988, 34; Garland 1992, 132.

39. On the history of Piraeus and its relation to Phaleron, see Garland 2001.

40. This is an inversion of de Polignac's mode, in which, as noted above, the polis articulates its periphery by locating cults at its borders.

41. On the Panathenaic procession, see Deubner 1932, 25–35; and Shear 2001, 122–167. On the processions of the City Dionysia, of which there were at least three, see Deubner 1932, 138–142; and Pickard-Cambridge 1968, 59–63. On the procession reenacting Dionysos' arrival and its relation to the Panathenaic procession, and for critique of de Polignac's argument that nonurban cults were unimportant to state formation in Athens, see Seaford 1994, 243–251. The roads of classical Athens have been studied in detail by Costaki 2006. My thanks to Leda Costaki for discussing with me the roads the Epidauria procession might have taken.

42. The Hierophant, as well as other priests and priestesses at Eleusis, were from the Eumolpid family. It was the Hierophant who, by definition, showed the holy things (*hiera*) to the initiates (Hesych. s.v. "ἱεροφάντες"), and he alone could enter the Anaktoron at Eleusis, where the holy things were kept (Aelian fr. 10). In later years, a separate vehicle was used to transport the interpreters, also members of the Eumolpid family, in the procession of the holy things from Eleusis to Athens (*Syll.*³ 587). See also Clinton 1974.

43. Clem. Al. *Protr.* 3.45.1; see also Cook 1995, 141. On the mythic war between Athens and Eleusis, and its symbolic articulation in Attic festivals, see Cook 1995, 134–145.

44. Athena as inventor of the chariot: *HHAph.* 12–13; Erichthonios as inventor: Marmor Parium 17–18. On Athena and the chariot, see also Yalouris 1950, 58–60. On apobatic competitions and the appearance of apobatai in the Parthenon frieze, see Shear 2001, 43–52; also Kyle 1992, 89–91, with n. 72 for bibliography on apobates. On the two- and four-horse chariot races, see Shear 2001, 283–293. Schultz (2007) argues that the west pediment of the Parthenon depicts Athena and Poseidon competing as apobatai. For ancient depictions of Panathenaic chariot races and apobates, see Kyle 1992, 89–93.

45. There are many parallels in literature and Attic ritual for Athena accompanying by chariot individuals whom she favors. See Connor 1987, 42–47.

46. My thanks to Leda Costaki for her many helpful observations on this leg of the procession. On the route and importance of the Street of the Tripods, see also Robertson 1998.

47. For bibliography, see Connor 1990, 10–11, followed by Anderson 2003, 178–184, who down-date the annexation to the last decade to the sixth century.

48. Fustel de Coulanges 1980, 201 (originally published in 1864).

49. Another piece of material evidence suggests Athenian interest in supporting the Epidaurian god: an Attic red-figure plate by the Meidias Painter, dated ca. 420 BC, depicts the personified Epidauros holding the infant Asklepios, with Eudaimonia seated to Asklepios' proper left. Given its date and subject matter, the plate may reflect Athens' efforts to promote the Epidaurian origins of its own, newly arrived Asklepios, while Eudaimonia's presence may point to Athens' good fortune in having received the god not only for his healing powers, as Lucilla Burn suggests (1987, 71), but also for his ability to forge an alliance between Athens and its recent enemy, Epidauros. On the plate, see also Shapiro 1993, 65–66; Stafford 2000, 155 with n. 30; illustrated in Burn 1987, pl. 46.

50. J.M. Hall 1999, 52.

Conclusions

1. Nutton (1986) urges caution in assuming that early Rome had only negative experiences with doctors. On early Roman perceptions of Greek medicine, see also Nutton 1993; von Staden 1996; Nutton 2004, 157–170, with references.

2. Only two other sanctuaries of Aesculapius are attested with certainty from Republican Italy. One is at Fregellae, dating to the second century BC; its excavators have noted Koan influence in its foundation and design. See Coarelli 1986; also Riethmüller 2005, vol. 2, 429–430 no. 579, for further references. The other is at Antium and is attested in literary sources (Val.Max. 1.8.2; De vir.ill. 22.3; Livy 43.6–7); see also Riethmüller 2005, vol. 2, 429 no. 575, for further evidence and references. The precise location of this sanctuary has not yet been determined. According to Valerius Maximus and the author of De viris illustribus, the sanctuary at Antium predates the arrival of Aesculapius in Rome.

3. By the fourth century BC various states had begun appealing to or thanking Asklepios for the safety of the state. On Athenian decrees thanking Asklepios and other gods for the health and safety of Athens, see Mikalson 1998, 42–44. Paeans from Epidauros and Delphi also ask the god to protect individual states (e.g., CA 132–136, 165–167).

4. Wickkiser 2003, chs. 7–9. This is a topic to which I hope to return in the future.

5. Wiseman 1995, 159.

6. Bowden 2005, 1–11; Lincoln 2003, esp. 51–61. As noted above in the Introduction, Bowden's book has been criticized for using extreme analogies.

7. "White coat hypertension" or the "white coat effect": e.g., Pickering et al. 1988; for a contrasting view, see Parati et al. 1998. The mute girl: IG IV² 1 123.1–3 = LiDonnici 1995 (C1). As noted by LiDonnici (esp. 117 n. 7, regarding this iama), the text of this inscription is heavily reconstructed.

8. For debate about the placebo effect, see Guess et al. 2002. Much has been written in recent years about the impact of medical trust on the healing process; see M.A. Hall 2002; Gatter 2004, with references. The complex relationship between religion and both medicine and science is still hotly debated—especially among the medical and scientific communities—as indicated by a spate of recent books on these subjects, such as Stephen J. Gould's Rocks of Ages: Science and Religion in the Fullness of Life (Ballantine, 1999) and Richard P. Sloan's Blind Faith: The Unholy Alliance of Religion and Medicine (St. Martin's Press, 2006).

Ackerknecht, E.H. 1946. "Natural Diseases and Rational Treatments in Primitive Medicine." *Bulletin of the History of Medicine* 19:467–497.

Alcock, S.E., and R. Osborne, eds. 1994. *Placing the Gods: Sanctuaries and Sacred Space in Ancient Greece.* Oxford.

Aleshire, S.B. 1989. *The Athenian Asklepieion: The People, Their Dedications, and the Inventories.* Amsterdam.

———. 1991. *Asklepios at Athens: Epigraphic and Prosopographic Essays on the Athenian Healing Cults.* Amsterdam.

———. 1992. "The Economics of Dedication at the Athenian Asklepieion," in Linders and Alroth, 85–99.

———. 1994. "Towards a Definition of 'State Cult' for Ancient Athens," in Hägg, 9–16.

Alfageme, R. 1995. "La médicine technique dans la comédie attique," in van der Eijk et al., 569–586.

Amundsen, D.W. 1977. "Images of the Physician in Classical Times." *Journal of Popular Culture* 11:643–655.

———. 1996. *Medicine, Society, and Faith in the Ancient and Medieval Worlds.* Baltimore.

Amundsen, D.W., and G.B. Ferngren. 1982. "Medicine and Religion: Pre-Christian Antiquity," in Marty and Vaux, 53–92.

Anderson, G. 2003. *The Athenian Experiment: Building an Imagined Political Community in Ancient Attica, 508–490 B.C.* Ann Arbor.

Arnott, G.W. 1979. *Menander.* Vol. 1. Loeb Classical Library. Cambridge, MA.

———. 2000. *Menander.* Vol. 3. Loeb Classical Library. Cambridge, MA.

Arnott, R. 1996. "Healing and Medicine in the Aegean Bronze Age." *Historical Review* 89:265–270.

———. 1999. "War Wounds and Their Treatment in the Aegean Bronze Age," in Laffineur, 499–506.

———. 2004. "Minoan and Mycenaean Medicine and Its Near Eastern Contacts," in Horstmanshoff and Stol, 153–173.

Asad, T. 1993. *Genealogies of Religion: Discipline and Reasons of Power in Christianity and Islam.* Baltimore.

Avalos, H. 1995. *Illness and Health Care in the Ancient Near East: The Role of the Temple in Greece, Mesopotamia, and Israel*. Atlanta.

———. 1999. *Health Care and the Rise of Christianity*. Peabody, MA.

Badian, E. 1987. "The Peace of Callias." *Journal of Hellenic Studies* 107:1–39.

———. 1993. *From Plataea to Potidaea: Studies in the History and Historiography of the Pentecontaetia*. Baltimore.

Bakker, E.J., ed. 1997. *Grammar as Interpretation: Greek Literature in Its Linguistic Contexts*. Mnemosyne supp. 171. Leiden.

Barron, J.P. 1964. "Religious Propaganda of the Delian League." *Journal of Hellenic Studies* 84:35–48.

Bates, D., ed. 1995. *Knowledge and the Scholarly Medical Traditions*. Cambridge.

Beard, M. 1992. "Frazer, Leach, and Virgil: The Popularity (and Unpopularity) of the Golden Bough," in *Comparative Studies in Society and Religion* 34.2:203–224.

Beard, M., J. North, and S. Price. 1998. *Religions of Rome*. Volume I: A History. Cambridge.

Behr, C.A. 1968. *Aelius Aristides and the Sacred Tales*. Amsterdam.

Bell, C. 1992. *Ritual Theory, Ritual Practice*. Oxford.

———. 1997. *Ritual: Its Perspectives and Dimensions*. Oxford.

Benedum, C. 1986. "Asklepios und Demeter." *Jahrbuch des Deutschen Archäologischen Instituts* 101:137–157.

Berger, E. 1970. *Das basler Arztrelief: Studien zum griechischen Grab- und Votivrelief um 500 v. Chr. und zur vorhippokratischen Medizin*. Basel.

Beschi, L. 1967/1968. "Il monumento di Telemachos, Fondatore dell'Asklepieion ateniese." *Annuario della Scuola Archeologica di Atene e delle Missioni Italiane in Oriente* 45–46 (ns 29/30): 381–436.

———. 1982. "Il rilievo di Telemachos ricompletato." *Αρχαιολογικά Ανάλεκτα εξ Αθηνών* 15.1:31–43.

———. 1985. "Rilievi attici del Museo Maffeiano," in Franzoni et al., 13–32.

———. 2002. "Culti stranieri e fondazioni private nell'Attica classica: Alcuni casi." *Annuario della Scuola Archeologica di Atene e delle Missioni Italiane in Oriente* 80:13–41.

Binder, J. 1984. "The West Pediment of the Parthenon: Poseidon," in Boegehold et al., 15–22.

Boedeker, D. 2007. "Athenian Religion in the Age of Pericles," in Samons, 46–69.

Boedeker, D., and K.A. Raaflaub, eds. 1998. *Democracy, Empire, and the Arts in Fifth-Century Athens*. Cambridge, MA.

Boegehold, A.L., et al. 1984. *Studies Presented to Sterling Dow on His Eightieth Birthday*. Greek, Roman, and Byzantine Monograph 10. Durham.

Bourgey, L., and J. Jouanna, eds. 1975. *La collection hippocratique et son rôle dans l'histoire de la médecine*. Leiden.

Bowden, H. 2005. *Classical Athens and the Delphic Oracle: Divination and Democracy*. Cambridge.

Bowersock, G.W. 1969. *Greek Sophists in the Roman Empire*. Oxford.

Bowie, A.M. 1993. *Aristophanes: Myth, Ritual and Comedy*. Cambridge.

Braarvig, J. 1999. "Magic: Reconsidering the Grand Dichotomy," in Jordan et al., 21–54.

Brock, R. 2000. "Sickness in the Body Politic: Medical Imagery in the Greek Polis," in Hope and Marshall, 24–34.

Broneer, O. 1943. "The Tent of Xerxes and the Greek Theater." *University of California Publications in Classical Archaeology* 1:305–312.

Bruit Zaidman, L., and P. Schmitt Pantel. 1992. *Religion in the Ancient Greek City.* Trans. P. Cartledge. Repr. Cambridge, 1994.

Brumfield, A.C. 1981. *The Attic Festivals of Demeter and Their Relation to the Agricultural Year.* Salem, NH.

Buchanan, S., ed. 1977. *The Portable Plato.* New York.

Burford, A. 1969. *The Greek Temple Builders at Epidauros: A Social and Economic Study of Building in the Asklepian Sanctuary, during the Fourth and Early Third Centuries B.C.* Toronto.

Burkert, W. 1983. *Homo Necans: The Anthropology of Ancient Greek Sacrificial Ritual and Myth.* Trans. Peter Bing. Berkeley.

———. 1985. *Greek Religion.* Trans. J. Raffan. Cambridge, MA.

———. 1987. *Ancient Mystery Cults.* Cambridge, MA.

———. 1992a. *The Orientalizing Revolution: Near Eastern Influence on Greek Culture in the Early Archaic Period.* Trans. M.E. Pinder and W. Burkert. Cambridge, MA.

———. 1992b. "The Formation of Greek Religion at the Close of the Dark Ages." *Studi italiani di filologia classica* 10:533–551.

———. 1994. "Olbia and Apollo of Didyma: A New Oracle Text," in Solomon, 49–60.

Burn, L. 1987. *The Meidias Painter.* Oxford.

Calame, C. 1996. *Thésée et l'imaginaire athénien: Légende et culte en Grèce antique.* 2nd edition. Lausanne.

Calder, W.H., III. 1971. "Stratonides Athenaios." *American Journal of Archaeology* 75: 325–329.

Camp, J.M. 1977. "The Water Supply of Ancient Athens from 3000 to 86 B.C." Ph.D. dissertation, Princeton University.

———. 1984. "Water and the Pelargikon," in Boegehold et al., 37–41.

———. 2001. *The Archaeology of Athens.* New Haven.

Cancik, H., and J. Rüpke, eds. 1997. *Römische Reichsreligion und Provinzialreligion.* Tübingen.

Cantor, D., ed. 2002. *Reinventing Hippocrates.* Aldershot.

Cavanaugh, M.B. 1996. *Eleusis and Athens: Documents in Finance, Religion and Politics in the Fifth Century B.C.* Atlanta.

Chantraine, P. 1956. *Études sur le vocabulaire grec.* Paris.

Chidester, D. 1996. *Savage Systems: Colonialism and Comparative Religion in Southern Africa.* Charlottesville.

Clinton, K. 1974. *The Sacred Officials of the Eleusinian Mysteries.* Philadelphia.

———. 1988. "Sacrifice at the Eleusinian Mysteries," in Hägg et al., 69–79.

———. 1992. *Myth and Cult: The Iconography of the Eleusinian Mysteries.* Stockholm.

———. 1993. "The Sanctuary of Demeter and Kore at Eleusis," in Marinatos and Hägg, 110–124.

———. 1994a. "The Epidauria and the Arrival of Asclepius in Athens," in Hägg, 17–34.

————. 1994b. "The Eleusinian Mysteries and Panhellenism in Democratic Athens," in Coulson et al., 161–172.

Coarelli, F., ed. 1986. *Fregellae: vol. 2. Il Santuario di Esculapio*. Rome.

Cohn-Haft, L. 1956. *The Public Physicians of Ancient Greece*. Northampton, MA.

Cole, T. 1991. *The Origins of Rhetoric in Ancient Greece*. Baltimore.

Collins, A.Y., and M.M. Mitchell, eds. 2001. *Antiquity and Humanity: Essays on Ancient Religion and Philosophy Presented to Hans Dieter Betz on His 70th Birthday*. Tübingen.

Comella, A. 2002. *I rilievi votivi greci di periodo arcaico e classico: Diffusione, ideologia, committenza*. Bari.

Connelly, J.B. 2007. *Portrait of a Priestess: Women and Ritual in Ancient Greece*. Princeton.

Connolly, A. 1998. "Was Sophocles Heroised as Dexion?" *Journal of Hellenic Studies* 118:1–21.

Connor, W.R. 1987. "Tribes, Festivals and Processions: Civic Ceremonial and Political Manipulation in Archaic Greece." *Journal of Hellenic Studies* 107:40–50.

————. 1990. "City Dionysia and Athenian Democracy," in Connor et al., 7–32.

Connor, W.R., et al. 1990. *Aspects of Athenian Democracy*. Classica et Mediaevalia, Dissertationes 11. Copenhagen.

Conrad, L.I., et al. 1995. *The Western Medical Tradition: 800 B.C.–A.D. 1800*. Cambridge.

Cook, E.F. 1995. *The Odyssey in Athens: Myths of Cultural Origins*. Ithaca.

Costaki, L. 2006. "The Intra Muros Road System of Ancient Athens." Ph.D. dissertation, University of Toronto.

Cotter, W. 1999. *Miracles in Greco-Roman Antiquity: A Sourcebook*. London.

Coulson, W.D.E., O. Palagia, T.L. Shear, Jr., H.A. Shapiro, and F.J. Frost, eds. 1994. *The Archaeology of Athens and Attica under the Democracy*. Proceedings of an international conference celebrating 2500 years since the birth of democracy in Greece, held at the American School of Classical Studies at Athens, December 4–6, 1992. Oxbow Monograph 37. Oxford.

Craik, E.M., ed. 1998. *Hippocrates, Places in Man*. Oxford.

Davies, J.K. 1971. *Athenian Propertied Families, 600–300 B.C.* Oxford.

Davies, J.P. 2004. *Rome's Religious History: Livy, Tacitus and Ammianus on Their Gods*. Cambridge.

Dean-Jones, L. 1995. "Autopsia, *Historia* and What Women Know: The Authority of Women in Hippocratic Gynaecology," in Bates, 41–59.

————. 2002. "Literacy and Orality in Classical Greek Medical Education." Paper delivered at the Fifth International Colloquium on Orality and Literacy, University of Melbourne, July 2002.

————. 2003. "Literacy and the Charlatan in Ancient Greek Medicine," in Yunis, 97–121.

Degrassi, D. 1986. "Il culto di Esculapio in Italia centrale durante il periodo repubblicano," in Coarelli, 145–152.

Demand, N. 1993. "Medicine and Philosophy: The Attic Orators," in Wittern and Pellegrin, 91–99.

de Polignac, F. 1995. *Cults, Territory, and the Origins of the Greek City-State*. Trans. J. Lloyd. Chicago.

Detienne, M. 1989. *Dionysus at Large*. Trans. A. Goldhammer. Cambridge, MA.

Deubner, L. 1932. *Attische Feste*. Repr. Berlin, 1956.

Dignas, B. 2007. "A Day in the Life of a Greek Sanctuary," in Ogden, 163–177.

Diller, H. 1970. *Hippokrates: Über die Umwelt (De aere aquis locis)*. Corpus medicorum graecorum I.1.2. Berlin.

Dillon, M.P.J. 1994. "The Didactic Nature of the Epidaurian Iamata." *Zeitschrift für Papyrologie und Epigraphik* 101:239–260.

———. 1997. *Pilgrims and Pilgrimage in Ancient Greece*. New York.

Dodds, E.R. 1951. *The Greeks and the Irrational*. Berkeley.

———. 1977. *Missing Persons: An Autobiography*. Oxford.

Dover, K. 1997. *The Evolution of Greek Prose Style*. Oxford.

Dunbar, N., ed. 1995. *Aristophanes: Birds*. Oxford.

Dunn, F. 2005. "On Ancient Medicine and Its Intellectual Context," in van der Eijk 2005a, ed., 49–67.

Edelstein, E.J., and L. Edelstein. 1945. *Asclepius: Collection and Interpretation of the Testimonies*. Repr. Baltimore, 1998.

Edelstein, L. 1943. *The Hippocratic Oath*. Baltimore.

Ehrhardt, N. 1989. "Apollon Ietros: Ein verschollener Gott Ioniens?" *Istanbuler Mitteilungen* 39:115–122.

Eliakes, K.M. 1992–1998. "Πρόταση για τη μορφή του αναθήματος του Τηλεμάχου Αχαρνέως." *Helios* 10–12:73–76.

Engelmann, H. 1975. *The Delian Aretalogy of Serapis*. Leiden.

Faraone, C., and D. Obbink, eds. 1991. *Magika Hiera: Ancient Greek Magic and Religion*. New York.

Farnell, L.R. 1896–1909. *Cults of the Greek States*. 5 vols. Oxford.

———. 1921. *Greek Hero Cults and Ideas of Immortality*. Oxford.

Feeney, D. 1998. *Literature and Religion at Rome: Cultures, Contexts, and Beliefs*. Cambridge.

Ferguson, W.S. 1944. "The Attic Orgeones." *Harvard Theological Review* 37:61–140.

Ferngren, G.B. 1992. "Early Christianity as a Religion of Healing." *Bulletin of the History of Medicine* 66:1–15.

Fiechter, E. 1930–1950. *Antike griechische Theaterbauten*. 9 vols. Stuttgart.

Fitzgerald, J.T., T.H. Olbricht, and L.M. White, eds. 2003. *Early Christianity and Classical Culture: Comparative Studies in Honor of Abraham J. Malherbe*. Novum Testamentum supp. 10. Leiden.

Foley, H.P., ed. 1994. *The Homeric Hymn to Demeter: Translation, Commentary, and Interpretive Essays*. Princeton.

Fornara, C.W., ed. 1983. *Archaic Times to the End of the Peloponnesian War*. Translated Documents of Greece and Rome. 2nd edition. Cambridge.

Forsén, B. 1996. *Griechische Gliederweihungen: Eine Untersuchung zu ihrer Typologie und ihrer religions- und sozialgeschichtlichen Bedeutung*. Helsinki.

Franzoni, L., et al. 1985. *Nuovi Studi Maffeiani: Atti del Convegno Scipione Maffei e il Museo Maffeiano, 18–19 November 1983*. Verona.

Fraser, R. 1990. *The Making of The Golden Bough: The Origins and Growth of an Argument*. New York.

Frazer, J.G. 1951. *The Golden Bough*. 3rd edition. 13 vols. London.

Frel, J. 1975. "The Telemachos Workshop." *J. Paul Getty Museum Journal* 2:15–16.

French, R., and F. Greenaway, eds. 1986. *Science in the Early Roman Empire: Pliny the Elder, His Sources and Influence.* London.

Friedländer, P., and H.B. Hoffleit. 1948. *Epigrammata: Greek Inscriptions in Verse from the Beginnings to the Persian Wars.* Berkeley.

Furley, W.R. 1993. "Besprechung und Behandlung: Zur Form und Funktion von ΕΠΩΙΔΑΙ in der griechischen Zaubermedizin," in Most et al., 80–104.

Fustel de Coulanges, N.D. 1980. *The Ancient City: A Study in the Religions, Laws, and Institutions of Greece and Rome.* Baltimore. (Originally published as *La cité antique: Étude sur le culte, le droit, les institutions de la Grèce et de Rome.* Paris, 1864.)

Gantz, T. 1993. *Early Greek Myth: A Guide to Literary and Artistic Sources.* Baltimore.

García Novo, E. 1995. "Structure and Style in the Hippocratic Treatise *Prorrheticon II*," in van der Eijk et al., 537–554.

Garland, R. 1984. "Religious Authority in Archaic and Classical Athens." *Annual of the British School at Athens* 79:75–123.

———. 1992. *Introducing New Gods: The Politics of Athenian Religion.* London.

———. 2001. *The Piraeus from the Fifth to the First Century BC.* 2nd edition. London.

Garofalo, I., et al., eds. 1999. *Aspetti della terapia nel Corpus Hippocraticum: Atti del IXe Colloque International Hippocratique (Pisa 25–29 settembre 1996).* Florence.

Gatter, R. 2004. "Faith, Confidence, and Health Care: Fostering Trust in Medicine through Law." *Wake Forest Law Review* 39:395–445.

Gebhard, E.R. 2001. "The Gods in Transit: Narratives of Cult Transfer," in Collins and Mitchell, 451–476.

Ghedini, F. 1980. *Sculture greche e romane del Museo civico di Padova.* Rome.

Girone, M. 1998. *Ἰάματα: Guarigioni miracolose di Asclepio in testi epigrafici.* Bari.

Goldhill, S. 1990. "The Great Dionysia and Civic Ideology," in Winkler and Zeitlin, 97–129.

Goldhill, S., and R. Osborne, eds. 2006. *Rethinking Revolutions through Ancient Greece.* Cambridge.

Gomme, A.W. 1945–1981. *A Historical Commentary on Thucydides.* 4 vols. Oxford.

Gordon, R. 1995. "The Healing Event in Graeco-Roman Folk-Medicine," in van der Eijk et al., 363–376.

Gorrini, M.E. 2001. "Gli eroi salutari dell'Attica." *Annuario della Scuola Archeologica di Atene e delle Missioni Italiane in Oriente* 79:299–315.

———. 2003. "Eroi salutari della Grecia continentale." Dissertation, L'Università degli Studi di Napoli "L'Orientale," Naples.

———. 2005. "The Hippocratic Impact on Healing Cults: The Archaeological Evidence in Attica," in van der Eijk 2005a, 135–156.

Graf, F. 1974. *Eleusis und die orphische Dichtung Athens in vorhellenistischer Zeit.* Berlin.

———. 1991. "Prayer in Magic and Religious Ritual," in Faraone and Obbink, 188–213.

———. 1992. "Heiligtum und Ritual: Das Beispiel der griechisch-römischen Asklepieia," in Schachter, 159–203.

———. 1996. "*Pompai* in Greece. Some Considerations about Space and Ritual in the Greek *Polis*," in Hägg, 55–65.

———. 1997. *Magic in the Ancient World*. Trans. F. Philip. Cambridge, MA.

———, ed. 1998. *Ansichten griechischer Rituale: Geburtstag-Symposium für Walter Burkert*. Castelen bei Basel, 15. bis 18. März 1996. Stuttgart.

Green, C.M.C. 2007. *Roman Religion and the Cult of Diana at Aricia*. Cambridge.

Grensemann, H. 1987. *Knidische Medizin Teil II: Versuch einer weiteren Analyse der Schicht A in den pseudohippokratischen Schriften* De natura muliebri und De muliebribus I und II. Stuttgart.

Guess, H.A., et al., eds. 2002. *The Science of the Placebo: Toward an Interdisciplinary Research Agenda*. London.

Habicht, C. 1969. *Die Inschriften des Asklepieions*. Vol. 8³. Berlin.

Hägg, R., ed. 1994. *Ancient Greek Cult Practice from the Epigraphical Evidence*. Proceedings of the Second International Seminar on Ancient Greek Cult, organized by the Swedish Institute at Athens, 22–24 November 1991. Stockholm.

———, ed. 1996. *The Role of Religion in the Early Greek Polis*. Proceedings of the Third International Seminar on Ancient Greek Cult, organized by the Swedish Institute at Athens, 16–18 October 1992. Stockholm.

———, ed. 1999. *Ancient Greek Hero Cult*. Proceedings of the Fifth International Seminar on Ancient Greek Cult, organized by the Department of Classical Archaeology and Ancient History, Göteborg University, 21–23 April 1995. Stockholm.

Hägg, R., N. Marinatos, and G.C. Nordquist, eds. 1988. *Early Greek Cult Practice*. Proceedings of the Fifth International Symposium at the Swedish Institute at Athens, 26–29 June 1986. Stockholm.

Hall, J.M. 1999. "Beyond the Polis: The Multilocality of Heroes," in Hägg, 49–59.

Hall, M.A. 2002. "Law, Medicine, and Trust." *Stanford Law Review* 55:463–501.

Hamilton, R. 2000. *Treasure Map: A Guide to the Delian Inventories*. Ann Arbor.

Hankinson, R.J. 1991. *Galen, On the Therapeutic Method: Books I and II*. Oxford.

———. 1992. "Doing Without Hypotheses: The Nature of Ancient Medicine," in López Férez, 55–67.

———. 1994. "Galen's Concept of Scientific Progress." *Aufstieg und Niedergang der römischen Welt* II.37.2: 1775–1789.

———. 1995. "Pollution and Infection: An Hypothesis Still-Born." *Apeiron* 28:25–65.

———. 1998a. *Cause and Explanation in Ancient Greek Thought*. Oxford.

———. 1998b. "Magic, Religion and Science: Divine and Human in the Hippocratic Corpus." *Apeiron* 31:1–34.

Harrison, T. 2006. "Religion and the Rationality of the Greek City," in Goldhill and Osborne, 124–140.

Hart, G.D. 2000. *Asclepius, the God of Medicine*. London.

Hausmann, U. 1948. *Kunst und Heiltum: Untersuchungen zu den griechischen Asklepiosreliefs*. Potsdam.

Hedrick, C.W., Jr. 1994. "Writing, Reading, and Democracy," in Osborne and Hornblower, 157–174.

Herzog, R. 1931. *Die Wunderheilungen von Epidauros: Ein Beitrag zur Geschichte der Medizin und der Religion*. Philologus supp. 22.3 Leipzig.

Hinnells, J.R., and R. Porter, eds. 1999. *Religion, Health, and Suffering*. New York.

Höckmann, U., and A. Krug, eds. 1977. *Festschrift für Frank Brommer*. Mainz.

Hogarth, D.G. 1908. *Excavations at Ephesus: The Archaic Artemisia*. London.

Holländer, E. 1912. *Plastik und Medizin*. Stuttgart.

Hölscher, T. 1991. "The City of Athens: Space, Symbol, Structure," in Molho et al., 355–380.

Holtzmann, B. 2003. *L'Acropole d'Athènes: Monuments, cultes et histoire du sanctuaire d'Athèna Polias*. Paris.

Hope, V.M., and E. Marshall, eds. 2000. *Death and Disease in the Ancient City*. London.

Horstmanshoff, H.F.J. 2004. "'Did the God Learn Medicine?' Asclepius and Temple Medicine in Aelius Aristides' *Sacred Tales*," in Horstmanshoff and Stol, 325–341.

Horstmanshoff, H.F.J., and M. Stol, eds. 2004. *Magic and Rationality in Ancient Near Eastern and Greco-Roman Medicine*. Studies in Ancient Medicine, vol. 27. Leiden.

Hubbard, T.K. 1992. "Remaking Myth and Rewriting History: Cult Tradition in Pindar's Ninth Nemean." *Harvard Studies in Classical Philology* 94:77–111.

Hurwit, J.M. 1999. *The Athenian Acropolis: History, Mythology, and Archaeology from the Neolithic Era to the Present*. Cambridge.

Isnardi Parente, M. 1966. *Techne: Momenti del pensiero greco da Platone ad Epicuro*. Florence.

Jameson, M.H. 1994. *A Greek Countryside: The Southern Argolid from Prehistory to the Present Day*. Stanford.

Janko, R. 1981. "Herbal Remedies at Pylos." *Minos* 17:30–34.

———. 1982. *Homer, Hesiod and the Hymns: Diachronic Development in Epic Diction*. Cambridge.

Jayne, W.A. 1925. *The Healing Gods of Ancient Civilizations*. New Haven.

Jeffrey, L.H. 1962. "The Inscribed Gravestones of Archaic Attica." *Annual of the British School at Athens* 57:115–153.

———. 1966. "Two Inscriptions from Iria." Αρχαιολογικόν Δελτίον 21A:18–24.

———. 1990. *Local Scripts of Archaic Greece: A Study of the Origin of the Greek Alphabet and Its Development from the Eighth to the Fifth Centuries B.C.* Rev. edition. Oxford.

Jensen, J., G. Hinge, P. Schultz, and B. Wickkiser, eds. Forthcoming. *Aspects of Ancient Greek Cult: Context—Ritual—Iconography*. Aarhus Studies in Mediterranean Antiquity 8. Aarhus.

Jones, D.W. 1999. *Peak Sanctuaries and Sacred Caves in Minoan Crete: Comparison of Artifacts*. Jonsered.

Jordan, D.R., H. Montgomery, and E. Thomassen, eds. 1999. *The World of Ancient Magic: Papers from the First International Samson Eitrem Seminar at the Norwegian Institute at Athens, 4–8 May 1997*. Bergen.

Jouanna, J. 1988. *Hippocrate. V.1: Des vents—De l'art*. Paris.

———. 1989. "Hippocrate de Cos et le sacré." *Journal des Savants*, January–June, 3–22.

———. 1990. *Hippocrate. II.1: L'Ancienne médecine*. Paris.

———. 1996. *Hippocrate. II.2: Airs, eaux, lieux*. Paris.

———. 1999. *Hippocrates*. Trans. M.B. DeBevoise. Baltimore.

———. 2003. *Hippocrate, II.3: La Maladie sacrée*. Paris.

Kallet, L. 1998. "Accounting for Culture in Fifth-Century Athens," in Boedeker and Raaflaub, 43–58.

———. 1999. "The Diseased Body Politic, Athenian Public Finance, and the Massacre at Mykalessos." *American Journal of Philology* 120:223–244.

Käppel, L. 1989. "Das Theater von Epidauros." *Jahrbuch des Deutschen Archäologischen Instituts* 104:83–106.

Kearns, E. 1989. *The Heroes of Attica*. London.

Kee, H.C. 1982. "Self-Definition in the Asclepius Cult," in Meyer and Sanders, 118–136.

———. 1983. *Miracle in the Early Christian World: A Study in Sociohistorical Method*. New Haven.

Keesling, C.M. 2005. "Misunderstood Gestures: Iconatrophy and the Reception of Greek Sculpture in the Roman Imperial Period." *Classical Antiquity* 24:41–79.

Kennedy, G.A. 1963. *The Art of Persuasion in Greece*. Princeton.

King, H. 1998. *Hippocrates' Woman: Reading the Female Body in Ancient Greece*. London.

———. 1999. "Comparative Perspectives on Medicine and Religion in the Ancient World," in Hinnells and Porter, 276–294.

———. 2002. "The Power of Paternity: The Father of Medicine Meets the Prince of Physicians," in Cantor, 21–36.

———, ed. 2005. *Health in Antiquity*. London.

———. 2006. "The Origins of Medicine in the Second Century AD," in Goldhill and Osborne, 246–263.

Körte, A. 1896. "Die Ausgrabungen am Westabhange der Akropolis IV." *Mitteilungen des Deutschen Archäologischen Instituts, Athenische Abteilung* 21:276–332.

Kosak, J.C. 2000. "*Polis nosousa*: Greek Ideas about the City and Disease in the Fifth Century BC," in Hope and Marshall, 35–54.

Kotansky, R. 1991. "Incantations and Prayers for Salvation on Inscribed Greek Amulets," in Faraone and Obbink, 107–137.

Krug, A. 1985. *Heilkunst und Heilkult: Medizin in der Antike*. Munich.

Kudlien, F. 1981. "Galen's Religious Belief," in Nutton, 117–130.

Kühlewein, H. 1894–1902. *Hippocratis Opera Omnia*. 2 vols. Leipzig.

Kullmann, W., and J. Althoff, eds. 1993. *Vermittlung und Tradierung von Wissen in der griechischen Kultur*. Tübingen.

Kutsch, F. 1913. *Attische Heilgötter und Heilheroen: Religionsgeschichtliche Versuche und Vorarbeiten* 12.3. Giessen.

Kyle, D.G. 1992. "The Panathenaic Games: Sacred and Civic Athletics," in Neils, 77–101.

Laffineur, R., ed. 1999. *Polemos: Le contexte guerrier en Égée à l'age du bronze. Aegeum 19*. 2 vols. Liège and Austin.

Lambrinoudakis, V. 1982. "Το ιερό του Απόλλωνος Μαλεάτα στην Επίδαυρο και η χρονολογία των κορινθιακών αγγείων." *Annuario della Scuola Archeologica di Atene e delle Missioni Italiane in Oriente* 44:49–55.

———. 2002. "Conservation and Research: New Evidence on a Long-living Cult, the Sanctuary of Apollo Maleatas and Asklepios at Epidauros," in Stamatopoulou and Yeroulanou, 213–224.

Lang, M.L. 1977. *Cure and Cult in Ancient Corinth: A Guide to the Asklepieion*. Princeton.

Langholf, V. 1990. *Medical Theories in Hippocrates: Early Texts and the "Epidemics."* Untersuchungen zur antiken Literatur und Geschichte 43. Berlin.

Laskaris, J. 1999. "Archaic Healing Cults as a Source for Hippocratic Pharmacology," in Garofalo et al., 1–12.

——. 2002. *The Art Is Long: On the Sacred Disease and the Scientific Tradition.* Leiden.

Lawton, C. 1995. *Attic Document Reliefs: Art and Politics in Ancient Athens.* Oxford.

——. Forthcoming. "Attic Votive Reliefs and the Peloponnesian War," in Palagia.

Lefantzis, M., and J. Jensen. Forthcoming. "The Athenian Asklepieion on the South Slope of the Akropolis I: Its Early Development from the Foundation in 420 to ca. 360 B.C.," in Jensen et al.

Lefkowitz, M.R. 1981. *The Lives of the Greek Poets.* London.

Ley, G. 1991. *A Short Introduction to the Ancient Greek Theater.* Chicago.

Lichtenthaeler, C. 1984. *Der Eid des Hippokrates: Ursprung und Bedeutung.* Cologne.

LiDonnici, L.R. 1995. *The Epidaurian Miracle Inscriptions: Text, Translation, and Commentary.* Society of Biblical Literature Texts and Translations 36; Graeco-Roman Religion Series 11. Atlanta.

Lincoln, B. 2003. *Holy Terrors: Thinking about Religion after September 11.* Chicago.

Linders, T., and B. Alroth, eds. 1992. *Economics of Cult in the Ancient Greek World: Proceedings of the Uppsala Symposium 1990. Boreas 21.* Uppsala.

Lloyd, G.E.R. 1970. *Early Greek Science: Thales to Aristotle.* New York.

——. 1979. *Magic, Reason, and Experience: Studies in the Origin and Development of Greek Science.* Cambridge.

——. 1983. *Science, Folklore and Ideology: Studies in the Life Sciences in Ancient Greece.* Cambridge.

——. 1987. *The Revolutions of Wisdom: Studies in the Claims and Practice of Ancient Greek Science.* Sather Classical Lectures, vol. 52. Berkeley.

——. 2003. *In the Grip of Disease: Studies in the Greek Imagination.* Oxford.

Longrigg, J. 1993. *Greek Rational Medicine: Philosophy and Medicine from Alcmaeon to the Alexandrians.* London.

Lopez, D.S., Jr. 1998. *Prisoners of Shangri-La: Tibetan Buddhism and the West.* Chicago.

López Férez, J.A., ed. 1992. *Tratados hipocráticos: Estudios acerca de su contenido, forma e influencia: Actas del VIIe Colloque international hippocratique, Madrid, 24–29 de septiembre de 1990.* Madrid.

Loraux, N. 1986. *The Invention of Athens: The Funeral Oration in the Classical City.* Trans. A. Sheridan. Cambridge, MA.

Lupu, E. 2005. *Greek Sacred Law: A Collection of New Documents (NGSL).* Leiden.

Majno, G. 1975. *The Healing Hand: Man and Wound in the Ancient World.* Cambridge, MA.

Mann, J. 2005. "Of Science, Skepticism, and Sophistry: The Pseudo-Hippocratic On the Art in Its Philosophical Context." Ph.D. dissertation, University of Texas at Austin.

Marinatos, N., and R. Hägg, eds. 1993. *Greek Sanctuaries: New Approaches.* London.

Mark, I. 1993. *The Sanctuary of Athena Nike in Athens: Architectural Stages and Chronology.* Hesperia supp. 26. Princeton.

Marshall, F.H. 1909. "Recent Acquisitions of the British Museum." *Journal of Hellenic Studies* 29:151–167.

Martin, D.B. 2004. *Inventing Superstition: From Hippocrates to the Christians.* Cambridge, MA.

Martin, R., and H. Metzger. 1976. *La religion grecque.* Paris.

Marty, M.E., and K.L. Vaux, eds. 1982. Health/Medicine and the Faith Traditions. Philadelphia.

Masuzawa, T. 2005. The Invention of World Religions: Or, How European Universalism Was Preserved in the Language of Pluralism. Chicago.

Melfi, M. 2003. "I santuari di Asclepio in Grecia." Ph.D. dissertation, University of Messina.

———. 2007. I santuari di Asclepio in Grecia. Vol. 1. Rome.

Meyer, B.F., and E.P. Sanders, eds. 1982. Self-Definition in the Greco-Roman World. Vol. 3, Jewish and Christian Self-Definition. Philadelphia.

Michaelis, A. 1876. "Bemerkungen zur Periegese der Akropolis von Athen." Mittheilungen des Deutschen Archaeologischen Institutes in Athen 1:275–307.

Mikalson, J.D. 1975. The Sacred and Civil Calendar of the Athenian Year. Princeton.

———. 1984. "Religion and the Plague in Athens, 431–23 B.C.," in Boegehold et al., 217–225.

———. 1998. Religion in Hellenistic Athens. Berkeley.

Miles, M.M. 1998. The City Eleusinion. Vol. 31 of The Athenian Agora: Results of Excavations Conducted by the American School of Classical Studies at Athens. Princeton.

Miller, M.C. 1997. Athens and Persia in the Fifth Century BC: A Study in Cultural Receptivity. Cambridge.

Miller, P.C. 1994. Dreams in Late Antiquity: Studies in the Imagination of a Culture. Princeton.

Mills, S. 1997. Theseus, Tragedy and the Athenian Empire. Oxford.

Mitchell-Boyask, R. 2007. "The Athenian Asklepieion and the End of the Philoctetes." Transactions of the American Philological Association 137:85–114.

Mitropoulou, E. 1975. A New Interpretation of the Telemachos Monument. Athens.

Molho, A., K. Raaflaub, and J. Emlen, eds. 1991. City-States in Classical Antiquity and Medieval Italy. Stuttgart.

Moore, T.J. 1998. The Theater of Plautus: Playing to the Audience. Austin.

Most, G., H. Petersmann, and A.M. Ritter, eds. 1993. Philanthropia kai Eusebeia: Festschrift für Albrecht Dihle zum 70. Geburtstag. Göttingen.

Murray, O., and S. Price, eds. 1990. The Greek City from Homer to Alexander. Oxford.

Musial, D. 1992. Le développement du culte d'Esculape au monde romain. Toruń.

Mylonas, G.E. 1960. "Ελευσίς και Διόνυσος." Αρχαιολογική Εφημερίς 68–118.

———. 1961. Eleusis and the Eleusinian Mysteries. Princeton.

Neils, J. 1987. The Youthful Deeds of Theseus. Rome.

———, ed. 1992. Goddess and Polis: The Panathenaic Festival in Ancient Athens. Princeton.

———, ed. 1996. Worshipping Athena: Panathenaia and Parthenon. Madison.

Nielsen, I. 1999. Hellenistic Palaces: Tradition and Renewal. Aarhus.

Nilsson, M.P. 1951. Cults, Myths, Oracles, and Politics in Ancient Greece. Lund.

Noack, F. 1927. Eleusis: Die baugeschichtliche Entwicklung des Heiligtumes. Berlin.

Nongbri, B. 2008. "Dislodging 'Embedded' Religion: A Brief Note on a Scholarly Trope." Numen 55:440–460.

Nowicki, K. 1994. "Some Remarks on the Pre- and Protopalatial Peak Sanctuaries in Crete." Aegean Archaeology 1:31–48.

Nunn, J.F. 1996. Ancient Egyptian Medicine. London.

Nutton, V. 1973. "The Chronology of Galen's Early Career." Classical Quarterly 23: 158–171.

————, ed. 1981. *Galen: Problems and Prospects: A Collection of Papers Submitted at the 1979 Cambridge Conference.* London.

————. 1986. "The Perils of Patriotism: Pliny and Roman Medicine," in French and Greenaway, 30–58.

————. 1992. "Healers in the Medical Market place: Towards a Social History of Graeco-Roman Medicine," in Wear, 15–58.

————. 1993. "Roman Medicine: Tradition, Confrontation, Assimilation." *Aufstieg und Niedergang der römischen Welt* II.37.1:49–78.

————. 1995a. "Medicine in the Greek World, 800–50 BC," in Conrad et al., 11–38.

————. 1995b. "Roman Medicine, 250 BC–AD 200," in Conrad et al., 39–70.

————. 1995c. "The Medical Meeting Place," in van der Eijk et al., 3–25.

————. 2004. *Ancient Medicine.* London.

Oberhelman, S.M. 1993. "Dreams in Greco-Roman Medicine." *Aufstieg und Niedergang der römischen Welt* II.37.1:121–156.

Oehler, J. 1909. "Epigraphische Beiträge zur Geschichte des Aerztestandes." *Janus* 14:4–20.

Ogden, D., ed. 2007. *A Companion to Greek Religion.* Malden, MA.

Osborne, R.G. 1994. "Archaeology, the Salaminioi, and the Politics of Sacred Space in Archaic Attica," in Alcock and Osborne, 143–160.

Osborne, R., and S. Hornblower, eds. 1994. *Ritual, Finance, and Politics: Athenian Democratic Accounts, Presented to David Lewis.* Oxford.

Palagia, O. 1993. *The Pediments of the Parthenon.* Leiden.

————, ed. Forthcoming. *Athenian Art in the Peloponnesian War.* Cambridge.

Palagia, O., and A. Spetsieri-Choremi, eds. 2007. *The Panathenaic Games: Proceedings of an International Conference Held at the University of Athens, May 11–12, 2004.* Oxford.

Palinkas, J. 2008. "The Gateways of the City Eleusinion and the Sanctuary of Demeter and Kore at Eleusis." Ph.D. dissertation, Emory University.

Parati, G., et al. 1998. "Difference Between Clinic and Daytime Blood Pressure Is Not a Measure of the White Coat Effect." *Hypertension* 31:1185–1189.

Parke, H.W. 1977. *Festivals of the Athenians.* Ithaca.

Parker, R. 1983. *Miasma: Pollution and Purification in Early Greek Religion.* Oxford.

————. 1988. "Demeter, Dionysus and the Spartan Pantheon," in Hägg et al., 99–104.

————. 1996. *Athenian Religion: A History.* Oxford.

————. 2005. *Polytheism and Society at Athens.* Oxford.

Pearcy, L.T. 1992. "Diagnosis as Narrative in Ancient Literature." *American Journal of Philology* 113.4:595–616.

Peatfield, A.A.D. 1990. "Minoan Peak Sanctuaries: History and Society." *Opuscula Atheniensia* 18:117–131.

Penn, R.G. 1994. *Medicine on Ancient Greek and Roman Coins.* London.

Peppa-Papaioannou, E. 1985. "Πλήνια Ειδώλια από το Ιερό του Απόλωνα Μαλεάτα Επιδαυρίας." Ph.D. dissertation, University of Athens.

Perlman, P. 2000. *City and Sanctuary in Ancient Greece: The Theorodokia in the Peloponnese.* Göttingen.

Petrakos, V.C. 1968. Ο Ωρωπός και το ιερόν του Αμφιαράου. Athens.

————. 1997. Ο επιγραφές του Ωρωπού. Athens.

Petropoulou, A. 1981. "The 'Eparche' Documents and the Early Oracle at Oropos. *Greek, Roman and Byzantine Studies* 22:39–63.

Pickard-Cambridge, A. 1968. *The Dramatic Festivals of the Athenians.* 2nd edition. Oxford.

Pickering, T.G., et al. 1988. "How Common Is White Coat Hypertension?" *Journal of the American Medical Association* 259:225–228.

Pinault, J.R. 1992. *Hippocratic Lives and Legends.* Leiden.

Pirenne-Delforge, V., and E. Suárez de la Torre, eds. 2000. *Héros et heroines dans les mythes et les cultes grecs: Actes du Colloque organisé à l'Université de Valladolid du 26 au 29 mai 1999.* Kernos supp. 10. Liège.

Planeaux, C. 2000–2001. "The Date of Bendis' Entry into Attica." *Classical Journal* 96:165–183.

Pleket, H.W. 1983. "Arts en maatschappij in het oude Griekenland: De sociale status van de arts." *Tijdschrift voor Geschiedenis* 96:325–347.

————. 1995. "The Social Status of Physicians in the Greco-Roman World," in van der Eijk et al., 27–33.

Pollitt, J.J. 1990. *The Art of Ancient Greece: Sources and Documents.* Cambridge.

Potter, P., G. Maloney, and J. Desautels, eds. 1990. *La Maladie et les Maladies dans la Collection hippocratique: Acts du VIe Colloque international hippocratique.* Quebec.

Pouilloux, J. 1954. *La forteresse de Rhamnonte: Étude de topographie et d'histoire.* Paris.

Price, S. 1999. *Religions of the Ancient Greeks.* Cambridge.

Price, T.H. 1978. *Kourotrophos: Cults and Representations of the Greek Nursing Deities.* Leiden.

Prioreschi, P. 1992. "Did the Hippocratic Physician Treat Hopeless Cases?" *Gesnerus* 49:341–350.

Pritchett, W.K. 1995. *Thucydides' Pentekontaetia and Other Essays.* Amsterdam.

Privitera, G.A., ed. 1982. *Pindaro: Le Istmiche.* Milan.

Purday, K.M. 1987. "Minor Healing Cults within Athens and Its Environs." Ph.D. dissertation, University of Southampton.

Race, W.H., ed. 1997. *Pindar: Olympian Odes, Pythian Odes.* Cambridge, MA.

Ragep, F.J., and S.P. Ragep, eds. 1996. *Tradition, Transmission, Transformation.* Proceedings of two conferences on pre-modern science held at the University of Oklahoma. Leiden.

Rehm, R. 2002. *The Play of Space: Spatial Transformation in Greek Tragedy.* Princeton.

Renberg, G.H. 2006/2007. "Public and Private Places of Worship in the Cult of Asclepius at Rome." *Memoirs of the American Academy in Rome* 51/52:87–172.

Riethmüller, J.W. 1999. "Bothros and Tetrastyle: The Heroon of Asclepius in Athens," in Hägg, 123–143.

————. 2005. *Asklepios: Heiligtümer und Kulte.* Studien zu antiken Heiligtümern. 2 vols. Heidelberg.

Rivers, W.H.R. 1924. *Medicine, Magic, and Religion.* New York.

Robert, F. 1933. "L'édifice E d'Épidaure et la topographie du hiéron d'Asclepios." *Bulletin de Correspondance Hellénique* 57:380–393.

Robert, L. 1955. "Dédicaces et reliefs votifs." *Hellenica: Recueil d'épigraphie de numismatique et d'antiquités grecques* 10:5–166.

Robertson, N. 1998. "The City Center of Archaic Athens." *Hesperia* 67.3:283–302.

Robkin, A.L.H. 1979. "The Odeion of Perikles: The Date of Its Construction and the Periklean Building Program." *Ancient World* 2:3–12.

Roebuck, C. 1951. *The Asklepieion and Lerna.* Vol. 14 of *Corinth: Results of Excavations Conducted by the American School of Classical Studies at Athens.* Princeton.

Root, M.C. 1985. "The Parthenon Frieze and the Apadana Reliefs at Persepolis: Reassessing a Programmatic Relationship." *American Journal of Archaeology* 89:103–120.

Rudhardt, J. 1960. "La définition du délit d'impiété d'après la législation attique." *Museum Helveticum* 17:87–105.

Salazar, C.F. 2000. *The Treatment of War Wounds in Greco-Roman Antiquity.* Studies in Ancient Medicine 21. Leiden.

Samama, É. 2003. *Les médecins dans le monde grec: Sources épigraphiques sur la naissance d'un corps médical.* École pratique des Hautes Études, Sciences historiques et philologiques 3. Hautes études du monde gréco-romain 31. Geneva.

Samons, L.J., II, ed. 2007. *The Cambridge Companion to the Age of Pericles.* Cambridge.

Sandbach, F.H. 1977. *The Comic Theatre of Greece and Rome.* New York.

Scarborough, J. 1991. "The Pharmacology of Sacred Plants, Herbs, and Roots," in Faraone and Obbink, 138–174.

Schachter, A. 1981–. *Cults of Boiotia.* 4 vols. London.

———, ed. 1992. *Le sanctuaire grec: Huit exposés suivis de discussions. Vandœuvres-Genève, 20–25 août 1990.* Entretiens sur l'antiquité classique, vol. 37. Geneva.

Schiefsky, M.J. 2005. *Hippocrates. On Ancient Medicine.* Studies in Ancient Medicine 28. Leiden.

Schlaifer, R. 1940. "Notes on Athenian Public Cults." *Harvard Studies in Classical Philology* 51:241–260.

Schultz, P. 2001. "The Akroteria of the Temple of Athena Nike." *Hesperia* 70.1:1–47.

———. 2007. "The Iconography of the Athenian Apobates Race: Origins, Meanings, Transformations," in Palagia and Spetsieri-Choremi, 59–72.

———. N.d. "The Date and Allegory of the Nike Temple Parapet." Unpublished manuscript.

Schultz, P. and R. von den Hoff, eds. Forthcoming. *Structure, Image, Ornament: Architectural Sculpture in the Greek World.* Oxford.

Schwenk, C.J. 1985. *Athens in the Age of Alexander: The Dated Laws and Decrees of "the Lykourgan Era" 338-322 B.C.* Chicago.

Seaford, R. 1994. *Reciprocity and Ritual: Homer and Tragedy in the Developing City-State.* Oxford.

Semeria, A. 1986. "Per un censimento degli *Asklepieia* della Grecia continentale e delle isole." *Annali Della Scuola Normale Superiore di Pisa: Classe di Lettere e Filosofia,* ser. 3, no. 16:931–958.

Shapiro, H.A. 1989. *Art and Culture under the Tyrants in Athens.* Mainz.

———. 1993. *Personifications in Greek Art: The Representation of Abstract Concepts, 600-400 B.C.* Zurich.

———. 1996. "Democracy and Imperialism: The Panathenaia in the Age of Perikles," in Neils, 215–225.

Shear, J.L. 2001. "Polis and Panathenaia: The History and Development of Athena's Festival." Ph.D. dissertation, University of Pennsylvania.

Shelmerdine, C.W. 1985. *The Perfume Industry of Mycenaean Pylos*. Göteborg.

Sherwin-White, S.M. 1978. *Ancient Cos: An Historical Study from the Dorian Settlement to the Imperial Period*. Göttingen.

Sickinger, J.P. 1999. *Public Records and Archives in Classical Athens*. Chapel Hill.

Simms, R.R. 1985. "Foreign Religious Cults in Athens in the Fifth and Fourth Centuries B.C." Ph.D. dissertation, University of Virginia.

Simon, E. 1990. *Die Götter der Römer*. Munich.

Smith, J.Z. 1978. *Map Is Not Territory: Studies in the History of Religions*. Leiden.

———. 2004. *Relating Religion: Essays in the Study of Religion*. Chicago.

Smith, W.C. 1963. *The Meaning and End of Religion*. Repr. Minneapolis, 1991.

Smith, W.D. 1979. *The Hippocratic Tradition*. Ithaca.

———. 1990. *Hippocrates: Pseudepigraphic Writings*. Studies in Ancient Medicine 2. Leiden.

Snell, B., ed. 1971. *Tragicorum Graecorum Fragmenta*. Göttingen.

Sokolowski, F. 1969. *Lois sacrées des cités grecques*. Paris.

Solimano, G. 1976. *Asclepio: Le aree del mito*. Publicazioni dell'istituto di filologia classica e medievale 46. Genoa.

Solomon, J., ed. 1994. *Apollo: Origins and Influences*. Tucson.

Sourvinou-Inwood, C. 1988. "Further Aspects of Polis Religion." *Annali, Istituto orientale di Napoli: Archeologia e storia antica* 10:259–274.

———. 1990. "What Is Polis Religion?" in Murray and Price, 296–322.

———. 1994. "Something to Do with Athens: Tragedy and Ritual," in Osborne and Hornblower, 269–290.

Stafford, E. 2000. *Worshipping Virtues: Personification and the Divine in Ancient Greece*. London.

———. 2005. " 'Without You No One Is Happy': The Cult of Health in Ancient Greece," in King, 120–135.

Stamatopoulou, M. and M. Yeroulanou, eds. 2002. *Excavating Classical Culture: Recent Archaeological Discoveries in Greece*. Oxford.

Stavropoulos, S.G. 1996. *Τα Ασκληπιεία της Πελοποννήσου*. Patras.

Stengel, P. 1920. *Die griechischen Kultusaltertümer*. 3rd edition. Munich.

Stewart, A.F. 1985. "History, Myth, and Allegory in the Program of the Temple of Athena Nike, Athens." *Studies in the History of Art* 16:53–73.

Tambiah, S.J. 1990. *Magic, Science, Religion, and the Scope of Rationality*. Cambridge.

Temkin, O. 1991. *Hippocrates in a World of Pagans and Christians*. Baltimore.

Thivel, A. 1975. "Le 'divin' dans la *Collection hippocratique*," in Bourgey and Jouanna, 59–76.

———. 1981. *Cnide et Cos?: Essai sur les doctrines medicales dans la Collection hippocratique*. Paris.

Thomas, R. 1993. "Performance and Written Publication in Herodotus and the Sophistic Generation," in Kullmann and Althoff, 225–244.

Tinker, G.E. 1983. "Medicine and Miracle: A Comparison of Two Healing Types in the Late Hellenistic World." Ph.D. dissertation, University of California.

Tiussi, C. 1999. *Il culto di Esculapio nell'area nord-Adriatica*. Rome.

Tomlinson, R. A. 1983. *Epidauros*. Austin.

———. 1992. "Perachora," in Schachter, 321–351.

Travlos, I.N. 1971. *Pictorial Dictionary of Ancient Athens*. New York.

van Brock, N. 1961. *Recherches sur le vocabulaire médical du grec ancien: Soins et guérison*. Paris.

van der Eijk, P.J. 1990. "The 'Theology' of the Hippocratic Treatise *On the Sacred Disease*." *Apeiron* 23:87–119. Reprinted in van der Eijk 2005b (Ch. 1).

———. 1991. " 'Airs, Waters, Places' and 'On the Sacred Disease': Two Different Religiosities?" *Hermes* 119:168–176.

———. 1997. "Towards a Rhetoric of Ancient Scientific Discourse," in Bakker, 77–129.

———. 2004. "Divination, Prognosis and Prophylaxis: The Hippocratic Work 'On Dreams' (*De victu* 4) and Its Near Eastern Background," in Horstmanshoff and Stol, 187–218.

———, ed. 2005a. *Hippocrates in Context: Papers Read at the XIth International Hippocrates Colloquium, University of Newcastle upon Tyne, 27–31 August 2002*. Leiden.

———. 2005b. *Medicine and Philosophy in Classical Antiquity*. Cambridge.

van der Eijk, P.J., H.F.J. Horstmanshoff, and P.H. Schrijvers, eds. 1995. *Ancient Medicine in Its Socio-Cultural Context: Papers Read at the Congress Held at Leiden University, 13–15 April 1992*. Amsterdam.

van Straten, F. 1981. "Gifts for the Gods," in Versnel, 65–151.

Verbanck-Piérard, A. 2000. "Les héros guérisseurs: Des dieux comme les autres!" in Pirenne-Delforge and Suárez de la Torre, 281–332.

Versnel, H.S., ed. 1981. *Faith, Hope and Worship: Aspects of Religious Mentality in the Ancient World*. Leiden.

Vikela, E. 2006. "Healer Gods and Healing Sanctuaries in Attica: Similarities and Differences." *Archiv für Religionsgeschichte* 8:41–62.

Vlastos, G. 1949. "Religion and Medicine in the Cult of Asclepius: A Review Article." *Review of Religion* 13.3:269–290.

von Eickstedt, K.-V. 2001. Το Ασκληπιείον του Πειραιώς. Athens.

von Gall, H. 1977. "Das persische Königszelt und die Hallenarchitektur in Iran und Griechenland," in Höckmann and Krug, 119–132.

von Gerkan, A., and W. Müller-Wiener. 1961. *Das Theater von Epidauros*. Stuttgart.

von Staden, H. 1989. *Herophilus: The Art of Medicine in Early Alexandria*. Cambridge, MA.

———. 1990. "Incurability and Hopelessness: The Hippocratic Corpus," in Potter et al., 75–112.

———. 1996. "Liminal Perils: Early Roman Perceptions of Greek Medicine," in Ragep and Ragep, 369–418.

Walker, H.J. 1995. *Theseus and Athens*. Oxford.

Walker, S. 1979. "A Sanctuary of Isis on the South Slope of the Athenian Acropolis." *Annual of the British School at Athens* 74:243–257.

Ward, A.G., et al. 1970. *The Quest for Theseus*. London.

Wear, A., ed. 1992. *Medicine in Society*. Cambridge.

Weinreich, O. 1909. *Antike Heilungswunder: Untersuchungen zum Wunderglauben der Griechen und Römer.* Religionsgeschichtliche Versuche und Vorarbeiten 8.1. Giessen.

Westendorf, W. 1999. *Handbuch der altägyptischen Medizin.* 2 vols. Leiden.

Wickkiser, B.L. 2003. "The Appeal of Asklepios and the Politics of Healing in the Greco-Roman World." Ph.D. dissertation, University of Texas.

———. 2006. "Chronicles of Chronic Cases and Tools of the Trade at Asklepieia." *Archiv für Religionsgeschichte* 8:25–40.

———. Forthcoming. "Banishing Plague: Asklepios, Athens and the Great Plague Reconsidered," in Jensen et al.

Wiles, D. 1997. *Tragedy in Athens: Performance Space and Theatrical Meaning.* Cambridge.

Winkler, J.J. 1990. "The Ephebes' Song: *Tragoidia* and *Polis,*" in Winkler and Zeitlin, 20–62.

Winkler, J.J., and F.I. Zeitlin, eds. 1990. *Nothing to Do with Dionysus? Athenian Drama in Its Social Context.* Princeton.

Wiseman, T.P. 1995. *Remus: A Roman Myth.* Cambridge.

Wittern, R. 1979. "Die Unterlassung ärztlicher Hilfeleistung in der griechischen Medizin der klassischen Zeit." *Münchener medizinische Wochenschrift* 121:731–734.

Wittern, R., and P. Pellegrin. 1993. *Hippokratische Medizin und antike Philosophie.* Verhandlungen des VIII. Internationalen Hippokrates-Kolloquiums in Kloster Banz/Staffelstein vom 23. bis 28. September 1993. Hildesheim.

Woodman, A.J. 1988. *Rhetoric in Classical Historiography: Four Studies.* Portland, OR.

Woolf, G. 1997. "Polis-Religion and Its Alternatives in the Roman Provinces," in Cancik and Rüpke, 71–84.

Wycherley, R.E. 1978. *The Stones of Athens.* Princeton.

Wylock, M. 1972. "Les aromates dans les tablettes Ge de Mycènes." *Studi Micinei ed Egeo-Anatolici* 15:105–146.

Yalouris, N. 1950. "Athena als Herrin der Pferde." *Museum Helveticum* 7:19–101.

Yunis, H., ed. 2003. *Written Texts and the Rise of Literate Culture in Ancient Greece.* Cambridge.

Zeller, D. 2003. "The ΘΕΙΑ ΦΥΣΙΣ of Hippocrates and of other 'Divine Men'," in Fitzgerald et al., 49–69.

Zervos, S.G. 1932. *Les bistouris, les sondes et les curettes chirurgicales d'Hippocrate.* Athens.